THE FUNDAMENTAL PRINCIPLE

Do you read imperfectly? Can you observe then that when you look at the first word, or the first letter, of a sentence you do not see best where you are looking; that you see other words, or other letters, just as well as or better than the one you are looking at? Do you observe also that the harder you try to see the worse you see?

Now close your eyes and rest them, remembering some color, like black or white, that you can remember perfectly. Keep them closed until they feel rested, or until the feeling of strain has been completely relieved. Now open them and look at the first word or letter of a sentence for a fraction of a second. If you have been able to relax, partially or completely, you will have a flash of improved or clear vision, and the area seen best will be smaller.

After opening the eyes for this fraction of a second, close them again quickly, still remembering the color, and keep them closed until they again feel rested. Then again open them for a fraction of a second. Continue this alternate resting of the eyes and flashing of the letters for a time, and you may soon find that you can keep your eyes open longer than a fraction of a second without losing the improved vision.

If your trouble is with distant instead of near vision, use the same method with distant letters.

In this way you can demonstrate for yourself the fundamental principle of the cure of imperfect sight by treatment without glasses.

If you fail, ask someone with perfect sight to help you.

This Certificate

is given to __Emily A. Bates__ in grateful acknowledgment of a gift made to the people of the year A.D. 8113 and deposited in

Crypt of Civilization

at Oglethorpe University

near Atlanta, Georgia

along with photographs, books, motion picture films, and actual objects used in our daily life, all of which are to be preserved for posterity by:

Founder, Crypt of Civilization
President, Oglethorpe University

Archivist

OFFICE OF THE ARCHIVIST

Oglethorpe University

MANU DEI RESURREXIT

Good minds, good morals, good manners

Oglethorpe University, Ga.

October 18, 1938.

Mr. W. H. Bates, M.D.
210 Madison Ave.
New York, N. Y.

Dear Sir:

It gives me pleasure to advise you that our Advisory Board has selected your book, PERFECT SIGHT WITHOUT GLASSES, for inclusion in the Crypt of Civilization.

As you doubtless know practically every newspaper and magazine in America as well as radio broadcasting stations have carried and are carrying the stories of this remarkable project. The most authentic examples of the age in which we live and particularly the new chemical products which are so strikingly an example of our present civilization together with micro filmed books, models to scale and other objects are being assembled for deposit in the crypt to be sealed up for six thousand years. We would be pleased to have you present us with a copy of the latest edition of the above book. As it is necessary to destroy this in microfilming, an unbound but gathered copy of one with damaged cover will do equally as well as a perfect copy. The method of preservation is described in the enclosed bulletin.

Very truly yours,

T. K. Peters
OGLETHORPE UNIVERSITY
Director of Archives

* * * * * * *

Fac-simile of a letter from Oglethorpe University reprinted, together with the Certificate on the opposite page—by permission of the authorities of the University—as an acknowledgment of their kind regard for the work of the author.

FERDINAND VON ARLT
(1812-1887)

Distinguished Austrian ophthalmologist, Professor of Diseases of the Eye at Vienna, who believed for a time that accommodation was produced by an elongation of the visual axis, but finally accepted the conclusions of Cramer and Helmholtz.

The Cure of Imperfect Sight by Treatment Without Glasses

By
W. H. BATES, M.D.

Ninth Printing

WILDSIDE PRESS

On a tomb in the Church of Santa Maria Maggiore in Florence was found an inscription which read: "Here lies Salvino degli Armati, Inventor of Spectacles. May God pardon him his sins."

Nuova Enciclopedia Italiana, Sixth Edition.

TO THE MEMORY
OF THE
PIONEERS OF OPHTHALMOLOGY
THIS BOOK IS GRATEFULLY DEDICATED

PREFACE

This book aims to be a collection of facts and not of theories and insofar as it is, I do not fear successful contradiction. When explanations have been offered it has been done with considerable trepidation, because I have never been able to formulate a theory that would withstand the test of the facts either in my possession at the time, or accumulated later. The same is true of the theories of every other man, for a theory is only a guess, and you cannot guess or imagine the truth. No one has ever satisfactorily answered the question, "Why?" as most scientific men are well aware, and I did not feel that I could do better than others who had tried and failed. One cannot even draw conclusions safely from facts, because a conclusion is very much like a theory, and may be disproved or modified by facts accumulated later. In the science of ophthalmology, theories, often stated as facts, have served to obscure the truth and throttle investigation for more than a hundred years. The explanations of the phenomena of sight put forward by Young, von Graefe, Helmholtz and Donders have caused us to ignore or explain away a multitude of facts which otherwise would have led to the discovery of the truth about errors of refraction and the consequent prevention of an incalculable amount of human misery.

In presenting my experimental work to the public, I desire to acknowledge my indebtedness to Mrs. E. C. Lierman, whose co-operation during four years of arduous labor and prolonged failure made it possible to carry the work to a successful issue. I would be glad, further, to acknowledge my debt to others who aided me with suggestions, or more direct assistance, but am unable to do so, as they have requested me not to mention their names in this connection.

As there has been a considerable demand for the book from the laity, an effort has been made to present the subject in such a way as to be intelligible to persons unfamiliar with ophthalmology.

CONTENTS

PAGE

Preface vii

CHAPTER I

Introductory 1

    Prevalence of errors of refraction—Believed to be incurable and practically unpreventable—The eye regarded as a blunder of Nature—Facts which seem to justify this conclusion—Failure of all efforts to prevent the development of eye defects—Futility of prevailing methods of treatment—Conflict of facts with the theory of incurability of errors of refraction—These facts commonly explained away or ignored—The author unable to ignore them, or to accept current explanations— Finally forced to reject accepted theories.

CHAPTER II

Simultaneous Retinoscopy 17

    Retinoscopy the source of much of the information presented in this book—What the retinoscope is—Its possibilities not realized—Commonly used only under artificial conditions—Used by the author under the conditions of life on human beings and the lower animals— Thus many new facts were discovered—Conflict of these facts with accepted theories—Resulting investigations.

CHAPTER III

Evidence For the Accepted Theory of Accommodation 23

    Development of the theory—Behavior of the lens in accommodation as noted by Helmholtz—General acceptance of these observations as facts—Abandonment by Arlt of the true explanation of accommodation— Inability of Helmholtz to explain satisfactorily the supposed change of form in the lens—Question still unsettled—Apparent accommodation in lenseless eyes—Curious and unscientific theories advanced to account for it —Voluntary production of astigmatism—Impossibility of reconciling it with the theory of an inextensible eyeball.

CHAPTER IV

The Truth About Accommodation As Demonstrated
By Experiments on the Eye Muscles of Fish,
Cats, Dogs, Rabbits and Other Animals . . 38

Disputed function of the external muscles of the eyeball—Once regarded as possible factors in accommodation—This idea dismissed after supposed demonstration that accommodation depends upon the lens—Author's experiments demonstrate that accommodation
depends wholly upon these muscles—Accommodation
prevented and produced at will by their manipulation—
Also errors of refraction—The oblique muscles of accommodation—The recti concerned in the production of
hypermetropia and astigmatism—No accommodation
with one oblique cut, paralyzed, or absent—Paralysis of
accommodation in experimental animals accomplished
only by injection of atropine deep into the orbit, so as
to reach the oblique muscles — Accommodation unaffected by removal of the lens—Fourth cranial nerve
supplying superior oblique muscle a nerve of accommodation—Sources of error believed to have been eliminated in experiments.

CHAPTER V

The Truth About Accommodation As Demonstrated
By a Study of Images Reflected From the
Cornea, Iris, Lens and Sclera 54

Technique of Helmholtz defective—Image obtained
by his method on the front of the lens not sufficiently
distinct or stable to be measured—Failure of author to
get reliable image with various sources of light—Success with 1,000-watt lamp, diaphragm and condenser—
Image photographed—Images on cornea, iris, lens and
sclera also photographed — Results confirmed earlier
observations—Eyeball changes its shape during accommodation—Lens does not—Strain to see at near-point
produces hypermetropia—Strain to see at distance myopia—Method of obtaining the corneal image.

CHAPTER VI

The Truth About Accommodation As Demonstrated
By Clinical Observations 69

Results of experimental work confirmed by clinical
observations—Atropine supposed to prevent accommodation—Conflict of facts with this theory—Normal accommodation observed in eyes under influence of atro-

PAGE

pine for long periods—Evidence of these cases against accepted theories overwhelming—Cases of accommodation in lenseless eyes observed by author—Reality of the apparent act of accommodation demonstrated by the retinoscope—Evidence from the cure of presbyopia—Harmony of all clinical observations with views of accommodation and errors of refraction presented in this book.

CHAPTER VII

The Variability of the Refraction of the Eye . . 75

Refractive states supposed to be permanent—Retinoscope demonstrates the contrary—Normal sight never continuous—Refractive errors always changing—Conditions which produce errors of refraction—Variability of refractive states the cause of many accidents—Also of much statistical confusion.

CHAPTER VIII

What Glasses Do to Us 81

The sins of Salvino degli Armati reputed inventor of spectacles—How glasses harm the eyes—Sight never improved by them to normal—Always resented at first by the eye—Objects of vision distorted by them—Disagreeable sensations produced—Field of vision contracted—Difficulty of keeping the glass clean—Reflection of light from lenses annoying and dangerous—Inconvenience of glasses to physically active persons—Effect on personal appearance—No muscular strain relieved by them—Apparent benefits often due to mental suggestion—Fortunate that many patients refuse to wear them—At best an unsatisfactory substitute for normal sight.

CHAPTER IX

Cause and Cure of Errors of Refraction . . . 89

All abnormal action of external muscles of the eyeball accompanied by a strain to see — With relief of this strain all errors of refraction disappear—Myopia (or lessening of hypermetropia) associated with strain to see at the distance — Hypermetropia (or lessening of myopia) associated with strain to see at the near-point —Facts easily demonstrated by retinoscope—Effect of strain at the near-point accounts for apparent loss of accommodation in the lenseless eye—Mental origin of eyestrain—Accounts for effect of civilization on the eye —Lower animals affected as man is—Remedy to get rid of mental strain—Temporary relaxation easy—Permanent relaxation may be difficult—Eyes not rested by sleep or tired by use—Rested only by resting the mind —Time required for a cure.

CHAPTER X

Strain   106

Foundation of the strain to see—Act of seeing passive —Same true of action of all sensory nerves—Their efficiency impaired when made the subject of effort—The mind the source of all such efforts brought to bear upon the eye—Mental strain of any kind produces eyestrain— This strain takes many forms—Results in production of many abnormal conditions — Circulation disturbed by strain—Normal circulation restored by mental control— Thus errors of refraction and other abnormal conditions are cured.

CHAPTER XI

Central Fixation   114

The center of sight—The eye normally sees one part of everything it looks at best—Central fixation lost in all abnormal conditions of the eye—Cause of mental strain —With central fixation the eye is perfectly at rest—Can be used indefinitely without fatigue—Open and quiet— No wrinkles or dark circles around it—Visual axes parallel—With eccentric fixation the contrary is the case— Eccentric fixation cured by any method that relieves strain—Limits of vision determined by central fixation— Organic diseases relieved or cured by it—No limit can be set to its possibilities—Relation to general efficiency and general health.

CHAPTER XII

Palming   123

Relaxation with the eyes shut—With light excluded by palms of the hands (palming)—Evidence of complete relaxation in palming—Of incomplete relaxation—Difficulties of palming—How dealt with—Futility of effort— All the sensory nerves relaxed by successful palming— Pain relieved in all parts of the body—Patients who succeed at once are quickly cured—A minority not helped and should try other methods.

CHAPTER XIII

PAGE

Memory As an Aid to Vision 136

Memory a test of relaxation—Memory of black most suitable for the purpose—Application of this fact to treatment of functional eye troubles—Sensation not a reliable index of strain—Memory of black is—Enables the patient to avoid conditions that produce strain—Conditions favorable to memory—Retention of memory under unfavorable conditions—Quick cures by its aid—A great held to other mental processes— Tests of a perfect memory.

CHAPTER XIV

Imagination As an Aid to Vision 148

Retinal impressions interpreted by the mind—Memory or imagination normally used as an aid to sight—In imperfect sight the mind adds imperfections to the imperfect retinal image—Only a small part of the phenomena of refractive errors accounted for by the inaccuracy of the focus—Difference between the photographic picture when the camera is out of focus and the visual impressions of the mind when the eye is out of focus—Patients helped by understanding of this fact—Dependence of imagination upon memory—Coincidence of both with sight—Perfect imagination dependent upon relaxation—Therefore imagination cures—Method of using it for this purpose—Remarkable cures effected by it.

CHAPTER XV

Shifting and Swinging 159

Apparent movement of objects regarded with normal vision—Due to unconscious shifting of the eye—Impossibility of fixing a point for an appreciable length of time—lowering of vision by attempt to do so—Inconspicuousness of normal shifting—Its incredible rapidity—Staring an important factor in the production of imperfect sight—Tendency to stare corrected by conscious shifting and realization of apparent movement resulting from it—Conditions of success with shifting—The universal swing—Methods of shifting—Cures effected by this means.

CHAPTER XVI

The Illusions of Imperfect and of Normal Sight . . 172

Normal and abnormal illusions—Illusions of color—Of size—Of form—Of number—Of location—Of nonexistent objects—Of complementary colors—Of the

color of the sun—Blind spots—Twinkling stars—Cause
of illusions of imperfect sight—Voluntary production of
illusions—Illusions of central fixation—Normal illusions of color—Illusions produced by shifting—The up·
right position of objects regarded an illusion.

CHAPTER XVII

Vision Under Adverse Conditions a Benefit to the
Eye   183

Erroneous ideas of ocular hygiene—Conditions supposedly injurious may be a benefit to the eye—No foundation for universal fear of the light—Temporary discomfort but no permanent injury from it—Benefits of
sun-gazing—Of looking at a strong electric light—Not
light but darkness a danger to the eye—Sudden contrasts of light may be beneficial—Advantages of the
movies—Benefits of reading fine print—Reading in moving vehicles—In a recumbent posture—Vision under difficult conditions good mental training.

CHAPTER XVIII

Optimums and Pessimums   198

All objects not seen equally well when sight is imperfect—The eye has its optimums and pessimums—Some
easily accounted for — Others unaccountable — Familiar
objects optimums—Unfamiliar objects pessimums—Examples of unaccountable optimums and pessimums—
Variability of optimums and pessimums—Test card usually a pessimum—Pessimums which the patient is not
conscious of seeing—Pessimums associated with a strain
to see—How pessimums may become optimums.

CHAPTER XIX

The Relief of Pain and Other Symptoms by the Aid
of the Memory   202

No pain felt when the memory is perfect—All the
senses improved—Efficiency of the mind increased—
Operations performed without anaesthetics — Organic
disorders relieved—Facts not fully explained, but attested by numerous proofs—Possible relationship of the
principle involved to cures of Faith Curists and Christian Scientists.

CHAPTER XX   PAGE

Presbyopia: Its Cause and Cure   210

Failure of near vision as age advances—Supposed
normality of this phenomenon—Near-points expected
at different ages—Many do not fit this schedule—Some
never become presbyopic—Some retain normal vision
for some objects while presbyopic for others—First and
second of these classes of cases explained away or ignored—Third not heretofore observed—Presbyopia both
preventable and curable—Due to a strain to see at the
near-point—No necessary connection with age—Lens
may flatten and lose refractive power with advancing
years, but not necessarily—Temporary increase of presbyopia by strain at the near-point—Temporary relief by
closing the eyes or palming—Permanent relief by permanent relief of strain—How the author cured himself—
Other cures—Danger of putting on glasses at the presbyopic age—Prevention of presbyopia.

CHAPTER XXI

Squint and Amblyopia: Their Cause   .   .   . 221

Definition of squint—Theories as to its cause—Failure
of these theories to fit the facts—Failure of operative
treatment—State of the vision not an important factor—
Amblyopia ex anopsia—Association with squint not invariable—Supposed incurability—Spontaneous recovery
—Curious forms of double vision in squint—Invariable
association of squint and amblyopia with strain—Invariable relief following relief of strain—Voluntary production of squint by strain.

CHAPTER XXII

Squint and Amblyopia: Their Cure   .   .   . 227

Squint and amblyopia purely functional troubles—
Cured by any method that relieves strain—Relaxation
sometimes gained by voluntary increase of squint, or
production of other kinds—Remarkable cure effected in
this way—Strain relieved when patient is able to look
more nearly in the proper direction—Proper use of a
squinting eye encouraged by covering the good eye—
Children cured by use of atropine in one or both eyes—
Examples of cases cured by eye education.

CHAPTER XXIII   PAGE

Floating Specks: Their Cause and Cure . . . 236

    Floating specks a common phenomenon of imperfect sight—Their appearance and behavior—Theories as to their origin—A fruitful field for the patent-medicine business—Examples of the needless alarm they have caused—May be seen at times by any one—Simply an illusion caused by mental strain—This strain easily relieved—Illustrative cases.

CHAPTER XXIV

Home Treatment 242

    Many persons can cure themselves of defective sight—Only necessary to follow a few simple directions—How to test the sight—Children who have not worn glasses cured by reading the Snellen test card every day—Adults of the same class also benefited in a short time—Cases of adults and children who have worn glasses more difficult—Glasses must be discarded—How to make a test card—Need of a teacher in difficult cases—Qualifications of such teachers—Duty of parents.

CHAPTER XXV

Correspondence Treatment 246

    Correspondence treatment usually regarded as quackery—Impossible in the case of most diseases—Errors of refraction, not being diseases, admit of such treatment—Glasses successfully fitted by mail—Less room for failure in correspondence treatment of imperfect sight without glasses—Personal treatment more satisfactory, but not always available—Examples of cases cured by correspondence—Need for the co-operation of local practitioners in such treatment.

CHAPTER XXVI

The Prevention of Myopia in Schools: Methods
That Failed 251

    A much debated question—Literature on the subject voluminous and unreliable—All that is certainly known—Studies of Cohn—Confirmation of his observations by other investigators in America and Europe—Increase of myopia during school life unanimously attributed to near work—Inadequacy of this theory—Failure of preventive measures based upon it—New difficulties—The appeal to heredity—To natural adaptation—Objections to these views—Why all preventive measures have failed.

CHAPTER XXVII PAGE

The Prevention and Cure of Myopia and Other Errors of Refraction in Schools: A Method That Succeeded 259

Production of eyestrain by unfamiliar objects—Relief by familiar objects—Facts furnish the means of preventing and curing errors of refraction in schools—By this means children often gain normal vision with incredible rapidity—Results in schools of Grand Forks, N. D.; New York, and other cities—Improvement in mentality of children as eyesight improved—Reformation of truants and incorrigibles—Hypermetropia and astigmatism prevented and cured—Method succeeded best when teachers did not wear glasses—Success would be greater still under a more rational educational system—Prevalence of defective sight in American children—Its results —Practically all cases preventable and curable—Inexpensiveness of method recommended—Imposes no additional burden on the teachers—Cannot possibly hurt the children—Directions for its use.

CHAPTER XXVIII

The Story of Emily 270

Cure of defective eyesight by cured patients—Cures of fellow students, parents and friends by school children—Remarkable record of Emily—An illustration of the benefits to be expected from the author's method of preventing and curing imperfect sight in school children.

CHAPTER XXIX

Mind and Vision 274

Poor sight one of the most fruitful causes of retardation in schools—More involved in it than inability to see —The result of an abnormal condition of the mind— This cannot be changed by glasses—Memory among faculties impaired when vision is impaired—Memory of primitive man may have been due to the same cause as his keen vision—A modern example of primitive memory combined with primitive keenness of vision—Correspondence between differences in the faculty of memory and differences in visual acuity—Memory and eyesight of children spoiled by the same causes—Both dependent upon interest—Illustrative cases—All the mental faculties improved when vision becomes normal—Examples of such improvement—Relief of symptoms of insanity by eye education—Facts indicate a close relation between the problems of vision and those of education.

CHAPTER XXX   PAGE

Normal Sight and the Relief of Pain for Soldiers and
Sailors 284

Growth of militarism in the United States—Demand
for universal military training—Lack of suitable material for such training—Defective eyesight greatest impediment to the raising of an efficient army—None more
easily removed—Plan for correcting defects of vision
submitted to Surgeon General during the war—Not
acted upon—Now presented to the public with some
modifications—First requisite eye education in schools
and colleges—Eye education in training camps and at
the front also needed, even for those whose sight is
normal—How school system might be modified for military and naval use—Soldiers should not be allowed to
wear glasses—Importance of eye training to aviators—
Eye training for the relief of pain.

CHAPTER XXXI

Letters from Patients 290

Army officer cures himself—A teacher's experiences—
Mental effects of central fixation—Relief after twenty-
five years—Search for myopia cure rewarded—Facts
versus theories—Cataract relieved by central fixation.

CHAPTER XXXII

Reason and Authority 304

Inaccessibility of average mind to reason—Facts dis-
credited if contrary to authority—Patients discredit their
own experience under this influence—Cure of cataract
ignored by medical profession—Expulsion of author
from N. Y. Post Graduate Medical School for curing
myopia—Man not a reasoning being—Consequences to
the world.

CHAPTER XXXIII

How to Demonstrate the Fundamental Principles of
Treatment 312

Helpful Suggestions—The benefit of Palming—The
Effects of Light upon the Eyes and Suntreatment—Brain
tension relieved by improvement of Sight.

LIST OF ILLUSTRATIONS

Portrait of Ferdinand von Arlt.................Frontispiece

FIG.   PAGE

1. Patagonians   2
2. African Pigmies   3
3. Moros from the Philippines   6
4. Diagram of the hypermetropic, emmetropic and myopic
   eyeballs 11
5. The eye as a camera   13
6. Mexican Indians   15
7. Ainus, the aboriginal inhabitants of Japan.............   16
8. The usual method of using the retinoscope...........   18
9. Diagrams of the images of Purkinje   24
10. Diagram by which Helmholtz illustrated his theory of
    accommodation   27
11. Portrait of Thomas Young   28
12. Portrait of Hermann Ludwig Ferdinand von Helmholtz 31
13. Demonstration upon the eye of a rabbit that the infe-
    rior oblique muscle is an essential factor in accommoda-
    tion   40
14. Demonstration upon the eye of a carp that the superior
    oblique muscle is essential to accommodation   41
15. Demonstration upon the eye of a rabbit that the produc-
    tion of refractive errors is dependent upon the action of
    the external muscles   42
16. Demonstration upon the eye of a fish that the produc-
    tion of myopic and hypermetropic refraction is depend-
    ent upon the action of the extrinsic muscles   43
17. Production and relief of mixed astigmatism in the eye
    of a carp   45
18. Demonstration upon the eyeball of a rabbit that the
    obliques lengthen the visual axis in myopia   46
19. Demonstration upon the eye of a carp that the recti
    shorten the visual axis in hypermetropia.............   47
20. Lens pushed out of the axis of vision.................   48
21. Rabbit with lens removed   49
22. Experiment upon the eye of a cat, demonstrating that
    the fourth nerve, which supplies only the superior
    oblique muscle, is just as much a nerve of accommoda-
    tion as the third, and that the superior oblique muscle
    which it supplies is a muscle of accommodation.......50-51
23. Pithing a fish preparatory to operating upon its eyes..   52
24. Arrangements for photographing images reflected from
    the eyeball.......................................   55

FIG.   PAGE
25. Arrangements for holding the head of the subject
    steady while images were being photographed 56
26. Image of electric filament on the front of the lens.... 57
27. Images of the electric filament reflected simultaneously
    from the cornea and lens 58
28. Image of electric filament upon the cornea 60
29. Image of electric filament on the front of the sclera.... 62
30. Images on the side of the sclera 63
31. Multiple images upon the front of the lens............ 64
32. Reflection of the electric filament from the iris........ 65
33. Demonstrating that the back of the lens does not change
    during accommodation 67
34. Straining to see at the near-point produces hyperme-
    tropia 90
35. Myopia produced by unconscious strain to see at the
    distance is increased by conscious strain 91
36. Immediate production of myopia and myopic astigmat-
    ism in eyes previously normal by strain to see at the
    distance 92-93
37. Myopic astigmatism comes and goes according as the
    subject looks at distant objects with or without strain.. 94
38. Patient who has had the lens of the right eye removed
    for cataract produces changes in the refraction of this
    eye by strain 96-97
39. A family group strikingly illustrating the effect of the
    mind upon the vision 99
40. Myopes who never went to school, or read in the Sub-
    way 100
41. One of the many thousands of patients cured of errors
    of refraction by the methods presented in this book.... 104
42. Palming 125
43. Patient with atrophy of the optic nerve gets flashes of
    improved vision after palming 127
44. Paralysis of the seventh nerve cured by palming 131
45. Glaucoma cured by palming 133
46. Woman with normal vision looking directly at the sun 187
47. Woman aged 37—child aged 4, both looking directly
    at the sun without discomfort 189
48. Focussing the rays of the sun upon the eye of a patient
    by means of a burning glass 191
49. Specimen of diamond type 195
50. Photographic type reduction 195
51. Operating without anaesthetics 204
52. Neuralgia relieved by palming and the memory of black. 207
53. Voluntary production of squint by strain to see........ 223
54. Case of divergent vertical squint cured by eye education 230
55. Temporary cure of squint by memory of a black period. 232
56. Face-rest designed by Kallmann, a German optician.... 254

THE CURE OF IMPERFECT SIGHT BY TREATMENT WITHOUT GLASSES

CHAPTER I

INTRODUCTORY

MOST writers on ophthalmology appear to believe that the last word about problems of refraction has been spoken, and from their viewpoint the last word is a very depressing one. Practically everyone in these days suffers from some form of refractive error. Yet we are told that for these ills, which are not only so inconvenient, but often so distressing and dangerous, there is not only no cure, and no palliative save those optic crutches known as eyeglasses, but, under modern conditions of life, practically no prevention.

It is a well-known fact that the human body is not a perfect mechanism. Nature, in the evolution of the human tenement, has been guilty of some maladjustments. She has left, for instance, some troublesome bits of scaffolding, like the vermiform appendix, behind. But nowhere is she supposed to have blundered so badly as in the construction of the eye. With one accord ophthalmologists tell us that the visual organ of man was never intended for the uses to which it is now put. Eons before there were any schools or printing presses, electric lights or moving pictures, its evolution was complete. In those days it served the needs of the human animal perfectly. Man was a hunter, a herdsman, a farmer, a fighter. He needed, we are told, mainly distant vision;

1

and since the eye at rest is adjusted for distant vision, sight is supposed to have been ordinarily as passive as the perception of sound, requiring no muscular action whatever. Near vision, it is assumed, was the exception,

Fig. 1. Patagonians

The sight of this primitive pair and of the following groups of primitive people was tested at the World's Fair in St. Louis and found to be normal. The unaccustomed experience of having their pictures taken, however, has evidently so disturbed them that they were all, probably, myopic when they faced the camera. (see Chapter IX.)

necessitating a muscular adjustment of such short duration that it was accomplished without placing any appreciable burden upon the mechanism of accommodation. The fact that primitive woman was a seamstress, an embroiderer, a weaver, an artist in all sorts of fine and beautiful work, appears to have been generally forgotten. Yet women living under primitive conditions have just as good eyesight as the men.

When man learned how to communicate his thoughts to others by means of written and printed forms, there came some undeniably new demands upon the eye, af-

Fig. 2. African Pigmies
They had normal vision when tested, but their expressions show that they could not have had it when photographed.

fecting at first only a few people, but gradually including more and more, until now, in the more advanced countries, the great mass of the population is subjected to their influence. A few hundred years ago even princes were not taught to read and write. Now we compel everyone to go to school, whether he wishes to or not, even the babies being sent to kindergarten. A generation or so ago books were scarce and expensive. To-day, by means of libraries of all sorts, stationary and traveling, they have been brought within the reach of practically everyone. The modern newspaper, with its endless columns of badly printed reading matter, was made possible only by the discovery of the art of manufacturing paper from wood, which is a thing of yesterday. The tallow candle has been but lately displaced by the various forms of artificial lighting, which tempt most of us to prolong our vocations and avocations into hours when primitive man was forced to rest, and within the last couple of decades has come the moving picture to complete the supposedly destructive process.

Was it reasonable to expect that Nature should have provided for all these developments, and produced an organ that could respond to the new demands? It is the accepted belief of ophthalmology to-day that she could not and did not,[1] and that, while the processes of civilization depend upon the sense of sight more than upon any other, the visual organ is but imperfectly fitted for its tasks.

There are a great number of facts which seem to justify this conclusion. While primitive man appears to have suffered little from defects of vision, it is safe to say that

---

[1] The unnatural strain of accommodating the eyes to close work (for which they were not intended) leads to myopia in a large proportion of growing children.—Rosenau: Preventive Medicine and Hygiene, third edition, 1917, p. 1093.

The compulsion of fate as well as an error of evolution has brought it about that the unaided eye must persistently struggle against the astonishing difficulties and errors inevitable in its structure, function and circumstance.—Gould: The Cause, Nature and Consequences of Eyestrain, Pop. Sci. Monthly, Dec., 1905.

With the invention of writing and then with the invention of the printing-press a new element was introduced, and one evidently not provided for by the process of evolution. The human eye which had been evolved for distant vision is being forced to perform a new part, one for which it had not been evolved, and for which it is poorly adapted. The difficulty is being daily augmented.—Scott: The Sacrifice of the Eyes of School Children, Pop. Sci. Monthly, Oct., 1907.

of persons over twenty-one living under civilized conditions nine out of every ten have imperfect sight, and as
the age increases the proportion increases, until at forty
it is almost impossible to find a person free from visual
defects.   Voluminous statistics are available to prove
these assertions, but the visual standards of the modern
army [1] are all the evidence that is required.

In Germany, Austria, France and Italy the vision with
glasses determines acceptance or rejection for military
service, and in all these countries more than six diopters[2]
of myopia are allowed, although a person so handicapped
cannot, without glasses, see anything clearly at more
than six inches from his eyes.   In the German Army a
recruit for general service is required—or was required
under the former government—to have a corrected vision
of 6/12 in one eye.   That is, he must be able to read
with this eye at six metres the line normally read at
twelve metres.   In other words, he is considered fit for
military service if the vision of one eye can be brought
up to one-half normal with glasses.   The vision in the
other eye may be minimal, and in the Landsturm one
eye may be blind.   Incongruous as the eyeglass seems
upon the soldier, military authorities upon the European
continent have come to the conclusion that a man with
6/12 vision wearing glasses is more serviceable than a
man with 6/24 vision (one-quarter normal) without
them.

In Great Britain it was formerly uncorrected vision
that determined acceptance or rejection for military service.   This was probably due to the fact that previous to
the recent war the British Army was used chiefly for

---

[1] Ford: Details of Military Medical Administration, published with the
approval of the Surgeon General, U. S. Army, second revised edition, 1918,
pp. 498-499.
[2] A diopter is the focussing power necessary to bring parallel rays to a
focus at one metre.

foreign service, at such distances from its base that there
might have been difficulty in providing glasses.   The
standard at the beginning of the war was 6/24 (uncorrected) for the better eye and 6/60 (uncorrected) for the

Fig. 3—Moros from the Philippines

With sight ordinarily normal all were probably myopic when
photographed except the one at the upper left whose eyes are
shut.

poorer, which was required to be the left.   Later, owing
to the difficulty of securing enough men with even this
moderate degree of visual acuity, recruits were accepted
whose vision in the right eye could be brought up to 6/12
by correction, provided the vision of one eye was 6/24
without correction.[1]

---

[1] Tr. **Ophth.** Soc. U. Kingdom, vol. **xxxviii**, 1918, pp. **130-131.**

Up to 1908 the United States required normal vision in recruits for its military service. In that year Bannister and Shaw made some experiments from which they concluded that a perfectly sharp image of the target was not necessary for good shooting, and that, therefore, a visual acuity of 20/40 (the equivalent in feet of 6/12 in metres), or even 20/70, in the aiming eye only, was sufficient to make an efficient soldier. This conclusion was not accepted without protest, but normal vision had become so rare that it probably seemed to those in authority that there was no use insisting upon it; and the visual standard for admission to the Army was accordingly lowered to 20/40 for the better eye and 20/100 for the poorer, while it was further provided that a recruit might be accepted when unable with the better eye to read all the letters on the 20/40 line, provided he could read some of the letters on the 20/30 line.[1]

In the first enrollment of troops for the European war it is a matter of common knowledge that these very low standards were found to be too high and were interpreted with great liberality. Later they were lowered so that men might be "unconditionally accepted for general military service" with a vision of 20/100 in each eye without glasses, provided that the sight of one eye could be brought up to 20/40 with glasses, while for limited service 20/200 in each eye was sufficient, provided the vision of one eye might be brought up to 20/40 with glasses.[2] Yet 21.68 per cent of all rejections in the first draft, 13 per cent more than for any other single cause, were for

---

[1] Harvard: Manual of Military Hygiene for the Military Services of the United States, published under the authority and with the approval of the Surgeon General, U. S. Army, third revised edition, 1917, p. 195.

[2] Standards of Physical Examination for the Use of Local Boards, District Boards, and Medical Advisory Boards under the Selective Service Regulations, issued through the office of the Provost Marshal General, 1918.

eye defects,[1] while under the revised standards these defects still constituted one of three leading causes of rejection. They were responsible for 10.65 per cent of the rejections, while defects of the bones and joints and of the heart and blood-vessels ran, respectively, about two and two and a half per cent higher.[2]

For more than a hundred years the medical profession has been seeking for some method of checking the ravages of civilization upon the human eye. The Germans, to whom the matter was one of vital military importance, have spent millions of dollars in carrying out the suggestions of experts, but without avail; and it is now admitted by most students of the subject that the methods which were once confidently advocated as reliable safeguards for the eyesight of our children have accomplished little or nothing. Some take a more cheerful view of the matter, but their conclusions are hardly borne out by the army standards just quoted.

For the prevailing method of treatment, by means of compensating lenses, very little was ever claimed except that these contrivances neutralized the effects of the various conditions for which they were prescribed, as a crutch enables a lame man to walk. It has also been believed that they sometimes checked the progress of these conditions; but every ophthalmologist now knows that their usefulness for this purpose, if any, is very limited. In the case of myopia[3] (shortsight), Dr. Sidler-Huguenin of Zurich, in a striking paper recently pub-

---

[1] Report of the Provost Marshal General to the Secretary of War on the First Draft under the Selective Service Act, 1917.

[2] Second Report of the Provost Marshal General to the Secretary of War on the Operations of the Selective Service System to December 20, 1918.

[3] From the Greek *myein*, to close, and *ops*, the eye; literally a condition in which the subject closes the eye, or blinks.

lished,[1] expresses the opinion that glasses and all methods now at our command are "of but little avail" in preventing either the progress of the error of refraction, or the development of the very serious complications with which it is often associated.

These conclusions are based on the study of thousands of cases in Dr. Huguenin's private practice and in the clinic of the University of Zurich, and regarding one group of patients, persons connected with the local educational institutions, he states that the failure took place in spite of the fact that they followed his instructions for years "with the greatest energy and pertinacity," sometimes even changing their professions.

I have been studying the refraction of the human eye for more than thirty years, and my observations fully confirm the foregoing conclusions as to the uselessness of all the methods heretofore employed for the prevention and treatment of errors of refraction. I was very early led to suspect, however, that the problem was by no means an unsolvable one.

Every ophthalmologist of any experience knows that the theory of the incurability of errors of refraction does not fit the observed facts. Not infrequently such cases recover spontaneously, or change from one form to another. It has long been the custom either to ignore these troublesome facts, or to explain them away, and fortunately for those who consider it necessary to bolster up the old theories at all costs, the rôle attributed to the lens in accommodation offers, in the majority of cases, a plausible method of explanation. According to this

---

[1] Archiv. f. Augenh, vol. lxxix, 1915, translated in Arch. Ophth., vol. xlv, No. 6, Nov., 1916.

theory, which most of us learned at school, the eye changes its focus for vision at different distances by altering the curvature of the lens; and in seeking for an explanation for the inconstancy of the theoretically constant error of refraction the theorists hit upon the very ingenious idea of attributing to the lens a capacity for changing its curvature, not only for the purpose of normal accommodation, but to cover up or to produce accommodative errors. In hypermetropia[1]—commonly but improperly called farsight, although the patient with such a defect can see clearly neither at the distance nor the nearpoint—the eyeball is too short from the front backward, and all rays of light, both the convergent ones coming from near objects, and the parallel ones coming from distant objects, are focussed behind the retina, instead of upon it. In myopia it is too long, and while the divergent rays from near objects come to a point upon the retina, the parallel ones from distant objects do not reach it. Both these conditions are supposed to be permanent, the one congenital, the other acquired. When, therefore, persons who at one time appear to have hypermetropia, or myopia, appear at other times not to have them, or to have them in lesser degrees, it is not permissible to suppose that there has been a change in the shape of the eyeball. Therefore, in the case of the disappearance or lessening of hypermetropia, we are asked to believe that the eye, in the act of vision, both at the near-point and at the distance, increases the curvature of the lens sufficiently to compensate, in whole or in part, for the flatness of the eyeball. In myopia, on the

---

[1] From the Greek *hyper*, over, *metron*, measure, and *ops*, the eye.

contrary, we are told that the eye actually goes out of its way to produce the condition, or to make an existing condition worse. In other words, the so-called "ciliary

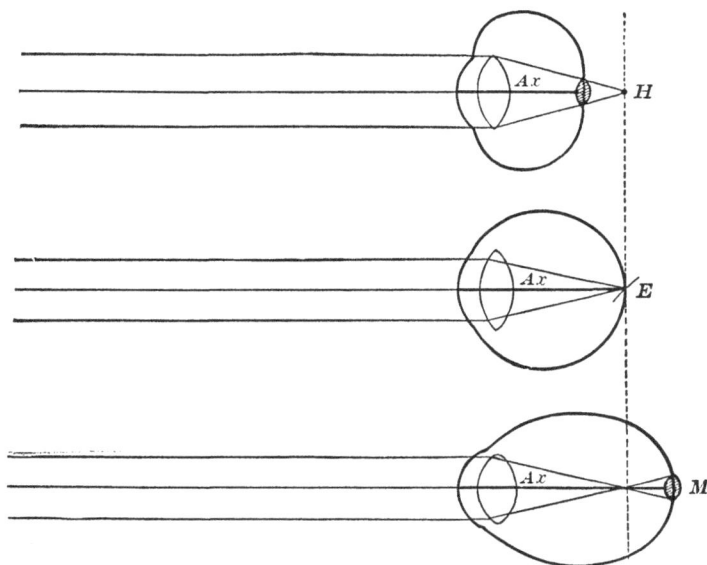

Fig. 4. Diagram of the Hypermetropic, Emmetropic and Myopic Eyeballs

H, hypermetropia; E, emmetropia; M, myopia; Ax, optic axis. Note that in hypermetropia and myopia the rays, instead of coming to a focus, form a round spot upon the retina.

muscle," believed to control the shape of the lens, is credited with a capacity for getting into a more or less continuous state of contraction, thus keeping the lens continuously in a state of convexity which, according to the theory, it ought to assume only for vision at the near-point. These curious performances may seem unnatural to the lay mind; but ophthalmologists believe the tendency to indulge in them to be so ingrained in the constitution of the organ of vision that, in the fitting of glasses, it is customary to instill atropine—the "drops" with which everyone who has ever visited an oculist is familiar—into the eye, for the purpose of paralyzing the ciliary muscle and thus, by preventing any change of curvature in the lens, bringing out "latent hypermetropia" and getting rid of "apparent myopia."

The interference of the lens, however, is believed to account for only moderate degrees of variation in errors of refraction, and that only during the earlier years of life. For the higher ones, or those that occur after forty-five years of age, when the lens is supposed to have lost its elasticity to a greater or less degree, no plausible explanation has ever been devised. The disappearance of astigmatism,[1] or changes in its character, present an even more baffling problem. Due in most cases to an unsymmetrical change in the curvature of the cornea, and resulting in failure to bring the light rays to a focus at any point, the eye is supposed to possess only a limited power of overcoming this condition; and yet astigmatism comes and goes with as much facility as do other errors of refraction. It is well known, too, that it can be produced voluntarily. Some persons can produce as much as three diopters. I myself can produce one and a half.

Examining 30,000 pairs of eyes a year at the New York Eye and Ear Infirmary and other institutions, I observed

---

[1] From the Greek *a*, without, and *stigma,* a point.

many cases in which errors of refraction either recovered spontaneously, or changed their form, and I was unable either to ignore them, or to satisfy myself with

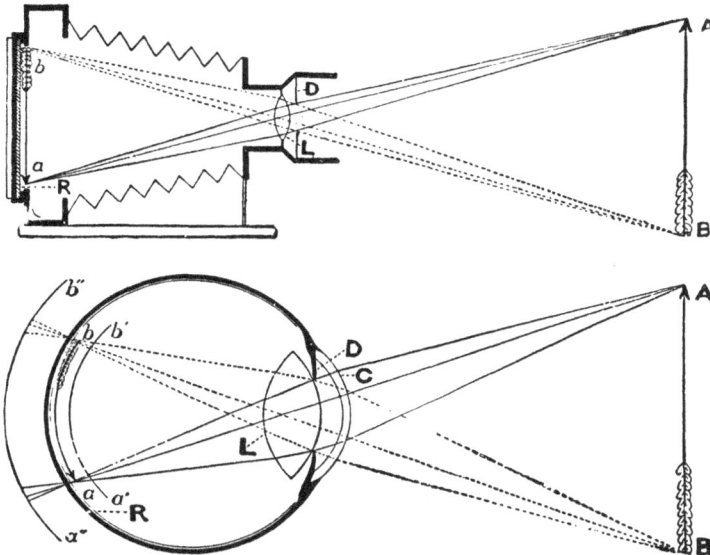

Fig. 5.   The Eye As a Camera

The photographic apparatus; D, diaphragm made of circular overlapping plates of metal by means of which the opening through which the rays of light enter the chamber can be enlarged or contracted; L, lens; R, sensitive plate (the retina of the eye ; AB, object to be photographed; ab, image on the sensitive plate.

The eye: C, cornea where the rays of light undergo a first refraction; D, iris (the diaphragm of the camera); L, lens, where the light rays are again refracted; R, retina of the normal eye; AB, object of vision; ab, image in the normal or emmetropic eye; a' b', image in the hypermetropic eye; a" b", image in the myopic eye.   Note that in a' b' and a" b", the rays are spread out upon the retina instead of being brought to a focus as in ab, the result being the formation of a blurred image.

the orthodox explanations, even where such explanations were available. It seemed to me that if a statement is a truth it must always be a truth. There can be no exceptions. If errors of refraction are incurable, they should not recover, or change their form, spontaneously.

In the course of time I discovered that myopia and hypermetropia, like astigmatism, could be produced at will; that myopia was not, as we have so long believed, associated with the use of the eyes at the near-point, but with a strain to see distant objects, strain at the near-point being associated with hypermetropia; that no error of refraction was ever a constant condition; and that the lower degrees of refractive error were curable, while higher degrees could be improved.

In seeking for light upon these problems I examined tens of thousands of eyes, and the more facts I accumulated the more difficult it became to reconcile them with the accepted views. Finally, about half a dozen years ago, I undertook a series of observations upon the eyes of human beings and the lower animals the results of which convinced both myself and others that the lens is not a factor in accommodation, and that the adjustment necessary for vision at different distances is affected in the eye, precisely as it is in the camera, by a change in the length of the organ, this alteration being brought about by the action of the muscles on the outside of the globe. Equally convincing was the demonstration that errors of refraction, including presbyopia, are due, not to an organic change in the shape of the eyeball, or in the constitution of the lens, but to a functional and therefore curable derangement in the action of the extrinsic muscles.

In making these statements I am well aware that I am controverting the practically undisputed teaching of ophthalmological science for the better part of a century;

Fig. 6. Mexican Indians

With normal sight when tested all the members of this primitive group are now either squinting or staring.

but I have been driven to the conclusions which they embody by the facts, and that so slowly that I am now surprised at my own blindness. At the time I was improving high degrees of myopia; but I wanted to be conservative, and I differentiated between functional myopia, which I was able to cure, or improve, and organic myopia, which, in deference to the orthodox tradition, I accepted as incurable.

Fig. 7. Ainus, the Aboriginal Inhabitants of Japan
All show signs of temporary imperfect sight

CHAPTER II

SIMULTANEOUS RETINOSCOPY

MUCH of my information about the eyes has been obtained by means of simultaneous retinoscopy. The retinoscope is an instrument used to measure the refraction of the eye. It throws a beam of light into the pupil by reflection from a mirror, the light being either outside the instrument—above and behind the subject—or arranged within it by means of an electric battery. On looking through the sight-hole one sees a larger or smaller part of the pupil filled with light, which in normal human eyes is a reddish yellow, because this is the color of the retina, but which is green in a cat's eye, and might be white if the retina were diseased. Unless the eye is exactly focussed at the point from which it is being observed, one sees also a dark shadow at the edge of the pupil, and it is the behavior of this shadow when the mirror is moved in various directions which reveals the refractive condition of the eye. If the instrument is used at a distance of six feet or more, and the shadow moves in a direction opposite to the movement of the mirror, the eye is myopic. If it moves in the same direction as the mirror, the eye is either hypermetropic or normal; but in the case of hypermetropia the movement is more pronounced than in that of normality, and an expert can usually tell the difference between the two states merely by the nature of the move-

Fig. 8. The Usual Method of Using the Retinoscope

The observer is so near the subject that the latter is made nervous, and this changes the refraction.

ment. In astigmatism the movement is different in different meridians. To determine the degree of the error, or to distinguish accurately between hypermetropia and normality, or between the different kinds of astigmatism, it is usually necessary to place a glass before the eye of the subject. If the mirror is concave instead of plane, the movements described will be reversed; but the plane mirror is the one most commonly used.

This exceedingly useful instrument has possibilities which have not been generally realized by the medical profession. Most ophthalmologists depend upon the Snellen[1] test card, supplemented by trial lenses, to determine whether the vision is normal or not, and to determine the degree of any abnormality that may exist. This is a slow, awkward and unreliable method of testing the vision, and absolutely unavailable for the study of the refraction of the lower animals, of infants, and of adult human beings under the conditions of life.

The test card and trial lenses can be used only under certain favorable conditions, but the retinoscope can be used anywhere. It is a little easier to use it in a dim light than in a bright one, but it may be used in any light, even with the strong light of the sun shining directly into the eye. It may also be used under many other unfavorable conditions.

It takes a considerable time, varying from minutes to hours, to measure the refraction with the Snellen test card and trial lenses. With the retinoscope, however, it can be determined in a fraction of a second. By the

---

[1] Herman Snellen (1835-1908). Celebrated Dutch ophthalmologist, professor of ophthalmology in the University of Utrecht and director of the Netherlandic Eye Hospital. The present standards of visual acuity were proposed by him, and his test types became the model for those now in use.

former method would be impossible, for instance, to get any information about the refraction of a baseball player at the moment he swings for the ball, at the moment he strikes it, and at the moment after he strikes it. But with the retinoscope it is quite easy to determine whether his vision is normal, or whether he is myopic, hypermetropic, or astigmatic, when he does these things; and if any errors of refraction are noted, one can guess their degree pretty accurately by the rapidity of the movement of the shadow.

With the Snellen test card and trial lenses conclusions must be drawn from the patient's statements as to what he sees; but the patient often becomes so worried and confused during the examination that he does not know what he sees, or whether different glasses make his sight better or worse; and, moreover, visual acuity is not reliable evidence of the state of the refraction. One patient with two diopters of myopia may see twice as much as another with the same error of refraction. The evidence of the test card is, in fact, entirely subjective; that of the retinoscope is entirely objective, depending in no way upon the statements of the patient.

In short, while the testing of the refraction by means of the Snellen test card and trial lenses requires considerable time, and can be done only under certain artificial conditions, with results that are not always reliable, the retinoscope can be used under all sorts of normal and abnormal conditions on the eyes both of human beings and the lower animals; and the results, when it is used properly, can always be depended upon. This means that it must not be brought nearer to the eye than six feet; otherwise the subject will be made nervous, the refraction, for reasons which will be explained later, will be changed, and no reliable observations will be possible.   In the case of animals it is often necessary to use it at a much greater distance.

For thirty years I have been using the retinoscope to study the refraction of the eye.   With it I have examined the eyes of tens of thousands of school children, hundreds of infants and thousands of animals, including cats, dogs, rabbits, horses, cows, birds, turtles, reptiles and fish.   I have used it when the subjects were at rest and when they were in motion—also when I myself was in motion; when they were asleep and when they were awake or even under ether and chloroform.   I have used it in the daytime and at night, when the subjects were comfortable and when they were excited; when they were trying to see and when they were not; when they were lying and when they were telling the truth; when the eyelids were partly closed, shutting off part of the area of the pupil, when the pupil was dilated, and also when it was contracted to a pin-point; when the eye was oscillating from side to side, from above downward and in other directions.   In this way I discovered many facts which had not previously been known, and which I was quite unable to reconcile with the orthodox teachings on the subject.   This led me to undertake the series of experiments already alluded to.   The results were in entire harmony with my previous observations, and left me no choice but to reject the entire body of orthodox teaching about accommodation and errors of refraction. But before describing these experiments I must crave the reader's patience while I present a résumé of the evidence upon which the accepted views of accommodation are based.   This evidence, it seems to me, is as strong an argument as any I could offer against the doctrine that the lens is the agent of accommodation, while an understanding of the subject is necessary to an understanding of my experiments.

CHAPTER III

EVIDENCE FOR THE ACCEPTED THEORY OF ACCOMMODATION

THE power of the eye to change its focus for vision at different distances has puzzled the scientific mind ever since Kepler[1] tried to explain it by supposing a change in the position of the crystalline lens. Later on every imaginable hypothesis was advanced to account for it. The idea of Kepler had many supporters. So also had the idea that the change of focus was effected by a lengthening of the eyeball. Some believed that the contractive power of the pupil was sufficient to account for the phenomenon, until the fact was established, by the operation for the removal of the iris, that the eye accommodated perfectly without this part of the visual mechanism. Some, dissatisfied with all these theories, discarded them all, and boldly asserted that no change of focus took place,[2] a view which was conclusively disproven when the invention of the ophthalmoscope made it possible to see the interior of the eye.

The idea that the change of focus might be brought about by a change in the form of the lens appears to have been first advanced, according to Landolt,[3] by the

---

[1] Johannes Kepler (1571-1630). German theologian, astronomer and physicist. Many facts of physiological optics were either discovered, or first clearly stated, by him.

[2] Donders: On the Anomalies of Accommodation and Refraction of the Eye. English translation by Moore, 1864, p. 10. Frans Cornelis Donders (1818-1889) was professor of physiology and ophthalmology at the University of Utrecht, and is ranked as one of the greatest ophthalmologists of all time.

[3] Edmund Landolt (1846-) Swiss ophthalmologist who settled in Paris in 1874, founding an eye clinic which has attracted many students.

23

Jesuit, Scheiner (1619).   Later it was put forward by
Descartes (1637).   But the first definite evidence in support of the theory was presented by Dr. Thomas Young
in a paper read before the Royal Society in 1800.[1]   "He
adduced reasons," says Donders, "which, properly under-

Fig. 9.   Diagrams of the Images of Purkinje

No. 1—Images of a candle: a, on the cornea; b, on the front
of the lens; c, on the back of the lens.

No. 2.—Images of lights shining through rectangular openings
in a screen while the eye is at rest (R) and during accommodation (A): a, on the cornea; b, on the front of the lens; c, on the
back of the lens (after Helmholtz).

Note that in No. 2, A, the central images are smaller and have
approached each other, a change which, if actually took place,
would indicate an increase of curvature in the front of the lens
during accommodation.

stood, should be taken as positive proofs."[2]   At the time,
however, they attracted little attention.

About half a century later it occurred to Maximilian
Langenbeck[3] to seek light on the problem by the aid of

---

[1] On the Mechanism of the Eye, Phil. Tr. Roy. Soc., London, 1801.
[2] On the Anomalies of Accommodation and Refraction of the Eye, pp. 10-11.
[3] Maximilian Adolf Langenbeck (1818-1877). Professor of anatomy, surgery
and ophthalmology at Göttingen, from 1846 to 1851.   Later settled in Hanover.

what are known as the images of Purkinje.[1] If a small bright light, usually a candle, is held in front of and a little to one side of the eye, three images are seen: one bright and upright; another large, but less bright, and also upright; and a third small, bright and inverted. The first comes from the cornea, the transparent covering of the iris and pupil, and the other two from the lens, the upright one from the front and the inverted one from the back.   The corneal reflection was known to the ancients, although its origin was not discovered till later; but the two reflections from the lens were first observed in 1823 by Purkinje; whence the trio of images is now associated with his name.   Langenbeck examined these images with the naked eye, and reached the conclusion that during accommodation the middle one became smaller than when the eye was at rest.   And since an image reflected from a convex surface is diminished in proportion to the convexity of that surface, he concluded that the front of the lens became more convex when the eye adjusted itself for near vision.   Donders repeated the experiments of Langenbeck, but was unable to make any satisfactory observations.   He predicted, however, that if the images were examined with a magnifier they would "show with certainty" whether the form of the lens changed during accommodation. Cramer,[2] acting on this suggestion, examined the images as magnified from ten to twenty times, and thus convinced himself that the one reflected from the front of the lens became considerably smaller during accommodation.

---

[1] Johannes Evangelista von Purkinje (1787-1869).   Professor of physiology at Breslau and Prague, and the discoverer of many important physiological facts.
[2] Antonie C. Cramer (1822-1855).   Dutch ophthalmologist.

Subsequently Helmholtz, working independently, made a similar observation, but by a somewhat different method.   Like Donders, he found the image obtained by the ordinary methods on the front of the lens very unsatisfactory, and in his "Handbook of Physiological Optics" he describes it as being "usually so blurred that the form of the flame cannot be definitely distinguished."[1] So he placed two lights, or one doubled by reflection from a mirror, behind a screen in which were two small rectangular openings, the whole being so arranged that the lights shining through the openings of the screen formed two images on each of the reflecting surfaces. During accommodation, it seemed to him that the two images on the front of the lens became smaller and approached each other, while on the return of the eye to a state of rest they grew larger again and separated. This change, he said, could be seen "easily and distinctly."[2] The observations of Helmholtz regarding the behavior of the lens in accommodation, published about the middle of the last century, were soon accepted as facts, and have ever since been stated as such in every text-book dealing with the subject.

"We may say," writes Landolt, "that the discovery of the part played by the crystalline lens in the act of accommodation is one of the finest achievements of medical physiology, and the theory of its working is certainly one of the most firmly established; for not only have "savans" furnished lucid and mathematical proofs of its correctness, but all other theories which have been advanced as explaining accommodation have been easily

---

[1] Handbuch der physiologischen Optik, edited by Nagel, 1909-11, vol. i, p. 121.
[2] Ibid, vol. i, p. 122.

and entirely overthrown. .. .. The fact that the eye is accommodated for near vision by an increase in the curvature of its crystalline lens, is, then, incontestably proved."[1]

Fig. 10.   Diagram by Which Helmholtz Illustrated His Theory of Accommodation

R is supposed to be the resting state of the lens, in which it is adjusted for distant vision.   In A the suspensory ligament is supposed to have been relaxed through the contraction of the ciliary muscle, permitting the lens to bulge forward by virtue of its own elasticity.

"The question was decided," says Tscherning, "by the observation of the changes of the images of Purkinje during accommodation, which prove that accommodation is effected by an increase of curvature of the anterior surface of the crystalline lens."[2]

---

[1] The Refraction and Accommodation of the Eye and their Anomalies, authorized translation by Culver, 1886, p. 151.

[2] Physiologic Optics, authorized translation by Weiland, 1904, p. 163. Marius Hans Erik Tscherning (1854—) is a Danish ophthalmologist who for twenty-five years was co-director and director of the ophthalmological laboratory of the Sorbonne. Later he became professor of ophthalmology in the University of Copenhagen.

Fig. 11. Thomas Young (1773-1829)

English physician and man of science who was the first to
present a serious argument in support of the view that accommodation is brought about by the agency of the lens.

"The greatest thinkers," says Cohn, "have mastered a host of difficulties in discovering this arrangement, and it is only in very recent times that its processes have been clearly and perfectly set forth in the works of Sanson, Helmholtz, Brücke, Hensen and Völckers."[1]

Huxley refers to the observations of Helmholtz as the "facts of adjustment with which all explanations of that process must accord,"[2] and Donders calls his theory the "true principle of accommodation."[3]

Arlt, who had advanced the elongation theory and believed that no other was possible, at first opposed the conclusions of Cramer and Helmholtz,[4] but later accepted them.[5]

Yet in examining the evidence for the theory we can only wonder at the scientific credulity which could base such an important department of medical practice as the treatment of the eye upon such a mass of contradictions. Helmholtz, while apparently convinced of the correctness of his observations indicating a change of form in the lens during accommodation, felt himself unable to speak with certainty of the means by which the supposed change was effected,[6] and strangely enough the question is still being debated. Finding, as he states, "absolutely nothing but the ciliary muscle to which accommodation could be attributed,"[7] Helmholtz concluded that the changes which he thought he had observed in the curvature of the lens must be effected by the action of this muscle; but he was unable to offer any satisfac-

---

[1] The Hygiene of the Eye in Schools, English translation edited by Turnbull, 1886, p. 23. Hermann Cohn (1838-1906) was professor of ophthalmology in the University of Breslau, and is known chiefly for his contributions to ocular hygiene.

[2] Lessons in Elementary Physiology, sixth edition, 1872, p. 231.

[3] On the Anomalies of Accommodation and Refraction of the Eye, p. 13.

[4] Krankheiten des Auges, 1853-56, vol. iii, p. 219, et seq.

[5] Ueber die Ursachen und die Entstehung der Kurzsichtigkeit, 1876. Vorwort.

[6] Handbuch der physiologischen Optik, vol. i, pp. 124 and 145.

[7] Ibid, vol. i, p. 144.

tory theory of the way it operated to produce these results and he explicitly stated that the one he suggested possessed only the character of probability. Some of his disciples, "more loyal than the king," as Tscherning has pointed out, "have proclaimed as certain what he himself with much reserve explained as probable,"[1] but there has been no such unanimity of acceptance in this case as in that of the observations regarding the behavior of the images reflected from the lens. No one except the present writer, so far as I am aware, has ventured to question that the ciliary muscle is the agent of accommodation; but as to the mode of its operation there is generally felt to be much need for more light. Since the lens is not a factor in accommodation, it is not strange that no one was able to find out how it changed its curvature. It is strange, however, that these difficulties have not in any way disturbed the universal belief that the lens does change.

When the lens has been removed for cataract the patient usually appears to lose his power of accommodation, and not only has to wear a glass to replace the lost part, but has to put on a stronger glass for reading. A minority of these cases, however, after they become accustomed to the new condition, become able to see at the near-point without any change in their glasses. The existence of these two classes of cases has been a great stumbling block to ophthalmology. The first and more numerous appeared to support the theory of the agency of the lens in accommodation; but the second was hard to explain away, and constituted at one time, as Dr. Thomas Young observed, the "grand objection" to this idea. A number of these cases of apparent change of focus

---

[1] Physiologic Optics, p. 166.

Herman Ludwig Ferdinand von Helmholtz (1821-1894)
whose observations regarding the behavior of images reflected
from the front of the lens are supposed to have demonstrated
that the curvature of this body changes during accommodation

in the lensless eye having been reported to the Royal Society by competent observers, Dr. Young, before bringing forward his theory of accommodation, took the trouble to examine some of them, and considered himself justified in concluding that an error of observation had been made. While convinced, however, that in such eyes the "actual focal distance is totally unchangeable," he characterized his own evidence in support of this view as only "tolerably satisfactory." At a later period Donders made some investigations from which he concluded that "in aphakia[1] not the slightest trace of accommodative power remains."[2] Holmholtz expressed similar views, and von Graefe, although he observed a "slight residuum" of accommodative power in lensless eyes, did not consider it sufficient to discredit the theory of Cramer and Helmholtz. It might be due, he said, to the accommodative action of the iris, and possibly also to a lengthening of the visual axis through the action of the external muscles.[3]

For nearly three-quarters of a century the opinions of these masters have echoed through ophthalmological literature. Yet it is to-day a perfectly well-known and undisputed fact that many persons, after the removal of the lens for cataract, are able to see perfectly at different distances without any change in their glasses. Every ophthalmologist of any experience has seen cases of this kind, and many of them have been reported in the literature.

In 1872, Professor Förster of Breslau, reported[4] a

---

[1] Absence of the lens.

[2] On the Anomalies of Accommodation and Refraction of the Eye, p. 320.

[3] Archiv. f. Ophth., 1855, vol. ii, part 1, p. 187 et seq. Albrecht von Graefe (1828-1870) was professor of ophthalmology in the University of Berlin, and is ranked with Donders and Arlt as one of the greatest ophthalmologists of the nineteenth century.

[4] Klin. Montasbl. f. Augenh., Erlangen, 1872, vol. x, p. 39, et seq.

series of twenty-two cases of apparent accommodation in eyes from which the lens had been removed for cataract. The subjects ranged in age from eleven to seventy-four years, and the younger ones had more accommodative power than the elder. A year later Woinow of Moscow[1] reported eleven cases, the subjects being from twelve to sixty years of age. In 1869 and 1870, respectively, Loring reported[2] to the New York Ophthalmological Society and the American Ophthalmological Society the case of a young woman of eighteen who, without any change in her glasses, read the twenty line on the Snellen test card at twenty feet and also read diamond type at from five inches to twenty. On October 8, 1894, a patient of Dr. A. E. Davis who appeared to accommodate perfectly without a lens consented to go before the New York Ophthalmological Society. "The members," Dr. Davis reports,[3] "were divided in their opinion as to how the patient was able to accommodate for the near-point with his distance glasses on"; but the fact that he could see at this point without any change in his glasses was not to be disputed.

The patient was a chef, forty-two years old, and on January 27, 1894, Dr. Davis had removed a black cataract from his right eye, supplying him at the same time with the usual outfit of glasses, one to replace the lens, for distant vision, and a stronger one for reading. In October he returned, not because his eye was not doing well, but because he was afraid he might be "straining" it. He had discarded his reading glasses after a few weeks, and had since been using only his distance glasses. Dr.

---

[1] Archiv. f. Ophth., 1873, vol. xix, part 3, p. 107.

[2] Flint: Physiology of Man, 1875, vol. v, pp. 110-111.

[3] Davis: Accomodation in the Lensless Eye, Reports of the Manhattan Eye and Ear Hospital, Jan., 1895. The article gives a review of the whole subject.

Davis doubted the truth of his statements, never having seen such a case before, but found them, upon investigation, to be quite correct. With his lensless eye and a convex glass of eleven and a half diopters, the patient read the ten line on the test card at twenty feet, and with the same glass, and without any change in its position, he read fine print at from fourteen to eighteen inches. Dr. Davis then presented the case to the Ophthalmological Society but, as has been stated, he obtained no light from that source. Four months later, February 4, 1895, the patient still read 20/10 at the distance and his range at the near point had increased so that he read diamond type at from eight to twenty-two and a half inches. Dr. Davis subjected him to numerous tests, and though unable to find any explanation for his strange performances, he made some interesting observations. The results of the tests by which Donders satisfied himself that the lensless eye possessed no accommodative power were quite different from those reported by the Dutch authority, and Dr. Davis therefore concluded that these tests were "wholly inadequate to decide the question at issue." During accommodation the ophthalmometer[1] showed that the corneal curvature was changed and that the cornea moved forward a little. Under scopolamine, a drug sometimes used instead of atropine to paralyze the ciliary muscle (1/10 per cent solution every five minutes for thirty-five minutes, followed by a wait of half an hour), these changes took place as before; they also took place when the lids were held up. With the possible influence of lid pressure and of the ciliary muscle eliminated, therefore, Dr. Davis felt himself bound to conclude that the changes "must

---

[1] An instrument for measuring the curvature of the cornea.

have been produced by the action of the external muscles." Under scopolamine, also, the man's accommodation was only slightly affected, the range at the near-point being reduced only two and a half inches.

The ophthalmometer further showed the patient to have absolutely no astigmatism. It had showed the same thing about three months after the operation, but three and a half weeks after it he had four and a half diopters.

Seeking further light upon the subject Dr. Davis now subjected to similar tests a case which had previously been reported by Webster in the "Archives of Pediatrics."[1] The patient had been brought to Dr. Webster at the age of ten with double congenital cataract. The left lens had been absorbed as the result of successive needlings, leaving only an opaque membrane, the lens capsule, while the right, which had not been interfered with, was sufficiently transparent around the edge to admit of useful vision. Dr. Webster made an opening in the membrane filling the pupil of the left eye, after which the vision of this eye, with a glass to replace the lens, was about equal to the vision of the right eye without a glass. For this reason Dr. Webster did not think it necessary to give the patient distance glasses, and supplied him with reading glasses only—plane glass for the right eye and convex 16D for the left. On March 14, 1893, he returned and stated that he had been wearing his reading glasses all the time. With this glass it was found that he could read the twenty line of the test card at twenty feet, and read diamond type easily at fourteen inches. Subsequently the right lens was removed, after which no accommodation was observed in this eye. Two years later,

---

[1] Nov., 1893, p. 932.

March 16, 1895, he was seen by Dr. Davis, who found that the left eye now had an accommodative range of from ten to eighteen inches. In this case no change was observed in the cornea. The results of the Donders tests were similar to those of the earlier case, and under scopolamine the eye accommodated as before, but not quite so easily. No accommodation was observed in the right eye.

These and similar cases have been the cause of great embarrassment to those who feel called upon to reconcile them with the accepted theories. With the retinoscope the lensless eye can be seen to accommodate; but the theory of Helmholtz has dominated the ophthalmological mind so strongly that even the evidence of objective tests was not believed. The apparent act of accommodation was said not to be real, and many theories, very curious and unscientific, have been advanced to account for it. Davis is of the opinion that "the slight change in the curvature of the cornea, and its slight advancement observed in some cases, may, in those cases, account for some of the accommodative power present, but it is such a small factor that it may be elminated entirely, since in some of the most marked cases of accommodation in aphakial eyes no such changes have been observed."

The voluntary production of astigmatism is another stumbling block to the supporters of the accepted theories, as it involves a change in the shape of the cornea, and such a change is not compatible with the idea of an "inextensible"[1] eyeball. It seems to have given them less trouble, however, than the accommodation of the lensless

---

[1] Inasmuch as the eye is inextensible, it cannot adapt itself for the perception of objects situated at different distances by increasing the length of its axis, but only by increasing the refractive power of its lens.—De Schweinitz: Diseases of the Eye, eighth edition, 1916, pp. 35-36.

eye, because fewer of these cases have been observed and still fewer have been allowed to get into the literature. Some interesting facts regarding one have fortunately been given by Davis, who investigated it in connection with the corneal changes noted in the lensless eye. The case was that of a house surgeon at the Manhattan Eye and Ear Hospital, Dr. C. H. Johnson. Ordinarily this gentleman had half a diopter of astigmatism in each eye; but he could, at will, increase this to two diopters in the right eye and one and a half in the left. He did this many times, in the presence of a number of members of the hospital staff, and also did it when the upper lids were held up, showing that the pressure of the lids had nothing to do with the phenomenon. Later he went to Louisville, and here Dr. J. M. Ray, at the suggestion of Dr. Davis, tested his ability to produce astigmatism under the influence of scopolamine (four instillations, 1/5 per cent solution). While the eyes were under the influence of the drug the astigmatism still seemed to increase, according to the evidence of the ophthalmometer, to one and a half diopters in the right eye and one in the left. From these facts, the influence of the lids and of the ciliary muscle having been eliminated, Dr. Davis concluded that the change in the cornea was "brought about mainly by the external muscles." What explanation others offer for such phenomena I do not know.

CHAPTER IV

THE TRUTH ABOUT ACCOMMODATION AS DEMONSTRATED BY EXPERIMENTS ON THE EYE MUSCLES OF FISH, CATS, DOGS, RABBITS AND OTHER ANIMALS

THE function of the muscles on the outside of the eyeball, apart from that of turning the globe in its socket, has been a matter of much dispute; but after the supposed demonstration by Helmholtz that accommodation depends upon a change in the curvature of the lens, the possibility of their being concerned in the adjustment of the eye for vision at different distances, or in the production of errors of refraction, was dismissed as no longer worthy of serious consideration. "Before physiologists were acquainted with the changes in the dioptic system,"[1] says Donders, "they often attached importance to the external muscles in the production of accommodation. Now that we know that accommodation depends on a change of form in the lens this opinion seems scarcely to need refutation." He states positively that "many instances occur where the accommodation is wholly destroyed by paralysis, without the external muscles being the least impeded in their action," and also that "some cases are on record of paralysis of all or nearly all of the muscles of the eye, and of deficiency of the same, without diminution of the power of accommodation."[2]

If Donders had not considered the question settled, he

---

[1] The refractive system.
[2] On the Anomalies of Accommodation and Refraction of the Eye, p. 22.

might have inquired more carefully into these cases, and if he had, he might have been less dogmatic in his statements; for, as has been pointed out in the preceding chapter, there are plenty of indications that the contrary is the case. In my own experiments upon the extrinsic eye muscles of fish, rabbits, cats, dogs and other animals, the demonstration seemed to be complete that in the eyes of these animals accommodation depends wholly upon the action of the extrinsic muscles and not at all upon the agency of the lens. By the manipulation of these muscles I was able to produce or prevent accommodation at will, to produce myopia, hypermetropia and astigmatism, or to prevent these conditions. Full details of these experiments will be found in the "Bulletin of the New York Zoological Society" for November, 1914, and in the "New York Medical Journal" for May 8, 1915; and May 18, 1918; but for the benefit of those who have not the time or inclination to read these papers, their contents are summarized below.

There are six muscles on the outside of the eyeball, four known as the "recti" and two as the "obliques." The obliques form an almost complete belt around the middle of the eyeball, and are known, according to their position, as "superior" and "inferior." The recti are attached to the sclerotic, or outer coat of the eyeball, near the front, and pass directly over the top, bottom and sides of the globe to the back of the orbit, where they are attached to the bone round the edges of the hole through which the optic nerve passes. According to their position, they are known as the "superior," "inferior," "internal" and "external" recti. The obliques are the muscles of accommodation; the recti are concerned in the production of hypermetropia and astigmatism.

In some cases one of the obliques is absent or rudimentary, but when two of these muscles were present and active, accommodation, as measured by the objective test

Fig. 13.   Demonstration Upon the Eye of a Rabbit that the Inferior Oblique Muscle is an Essential Factor in Accommodation

No. 1.—The inferior oblique muscle has been exposed and two sutures are attached to it.   Electrical stimulation of the eyeball produces accommodation, as demonstrated by simultaneous retinoscopy.

No. 2.—The muscle has been cut.   Electrical stimulation produces no accommodation.

No. 3.—The muscle has been sewed together. Electrical stimulation produces normal accommodation.

of retinoscopy, was always produced by electrical stimulation either of the eyeball, or of the nerves of accommodation near their origin in the brain.   It was also pro-

Fig. 14. Demonstration Upon the Eye of a Carp That the Superior Oblique Muscle Is Essential to Accommodation.

No. 1.—The superior oblique is lifted from the eyeball by two sutures, and the retinoscope shows no error of refraction. No. 2. —Electrical stimulation produces accommodation, as determined by the retinoscope. No. 3.—The muscle has been cut. Stimulation of the eyeball with electricity fails to produce accommodation. No. 4.—The divided muscle has been reunited by tying the sutures. Accommodation follows electrical stimulation as before.

duced by any manipulation of the obliques whereby their pull was increased. This was done by a tucking operation of one or both muscles, or by an advancement of the

Fig. 15.   Demonstration Upon the Eye of a Rabbit That the Production of the Refractive Errors Is Dependent Upon the Action of the External Muscles.   The String Is Fastened to the Insertion of the Superior Oblique and Rectus Muscles

No. 1.—Backward pull. Myopia is produced.

No. 2.—Forward pull. Hypermetropia is p r o - duced.

No. 3.—Upward pull in the p l a n e of the iris. Mixed astigmatism is produced.

point at which they are attached to the sclerotic. When one or more of the recti had been cut, the effect of operations increasing the pull of the obliques was intensified.

After one or both of the obliques had been cut across, or after they had been paralyzed by the injection of atropine deep into the orbit, accommodation could never be

Fig. 16. Demonstration Upon the Eye of a Fish That the Production of Myopic and Hypermetropic Refraction Is Dependent Upon the Action of the Extrinsic Muscles.

Suture tied to the insertion of the superior rectus muscle. By means of strong traction upon the suture the eyeball is turned in its socket, and by tying the thread to a pair of fixation forceps which grasp the lower jaw, it is maintained in this position. A high degree of mixed astigmatism is produced, as demonstrated by simultaneous retinoscopy. When the superior oblique is divided the myopic part of the astigmatism disappears, and when the inferior rectus is cut the hypermetropic part disappears, and the eye becomes normal—adjusted for distant vision—although the same amount of traction is maintained. It is evident that these muscles are essential factors in the production of myopia and hypermetropia.

produced by electrical stimulation; but after the effects of the atropine had passed away, or a divided muscle had been sewed together, accommodation followed electrical stimulation just as usual. Again when one oblique muscle was absent, as was found to be the case in a dogfish, a shark and a few perch, or rudimentary, as in all cats observed, a few fish and an occasional rabbit, accommodation could not be produced by electrical stimulation. But when the rudimentary muscle was strengthened by advancement, or the absent one was replaced by a suture whi h supplied the necessary countertraction, accommodation could always be produced by electrical stimulation.

After one or both of the oblique muscles had been cut, and while two or more of the recti were present and active,[1] electrical stimulation of the eyeball, or of the nerves of accommodation, always produced hypermetropia, while by the manipulation of one of the recti, usually the inferior or the superior, so as to strengthen its pull, the same result could be produced. The paralyzing of the recti by atropine, or the cutting of one or more of them, prevented the production of hypermetropic refraction by electrical stimulation; but after the effects of the atropine had passed away, or after a divided muscle had been sewed together, hypermetropia was produced as usual by electrical stimulation.

It should be emphasized that in order to paralyze either the recti muscles, or the obliques, it was found necessary to inject the atropine far back behind the eyeball with a hypodermic needle. This drug is supposed to paralyze the accommodation when dropped into the eyes of human

---

[1] In many animals, notably in rabbits, the internal and external recti are either absent or rudimentary, so that, practically, in such cases, there are only two recti, just as there are only two obliques. In others, as in many fish, the internal rectus is negligible.

beings or animals, but in all of my experiments it was found that when used in this way it had very little effect upon the power of the eye to change its focus.

Astigmatism was usually produced in combination

Fig. 17.

No. 1.—Production of mixed astigmatism in the eye of a carp by pulling strings attached to the conjunctiva in opposite directions. Note the oval shape of the front of the eyeball.

No. 2.—With the cutting of the strings the eyeball returns to its normal shape, and the refraction becomes normal.

with myopic or hypermetropic refraction.   It was also produced by various manipulations of both the oblique and recti muscles.   Mixed astigmatism, which is a combination of myopic with hypermetropic refraction, was

Fig. 18.   Demonstration Upon the Eyeball of a Rabbit That the Obliques Lengthen the Visual Axis in Myopia

R, rest. The eyeball is of normal length and emmetropic—that is, perfectly adjusted for distant vision. My, myopia. The pull of the oblique muscles has been strengthened by advancement, and the retinoscope shows that myopia has been produced. It can easily be noted that the eyeball is longer. It was impossible to avoid some movement of the head between the taking of the two pictures as a result of the manipulation of the strings, but the rule shows that the focus of the camera was not appreciably changed by such movements.

always produced by traction on the insertion of the superior or inferior rectus in a direction parallel to the plane of the iris, so long as both obliques were present and active; but if either or both of the obliques had been cut, the myopic part of the astigmatism disappeared. Similarly after the superior or the inferior rectus had been cut the hypermetropic part of the astigmatism disappeared. Advancement of the two obliques, with advancement of the superior and inferior recti, always produced mixed astigmatism.

Fig. 19. Demonstration Upon the Eye of a Carp That the Recti Shorten the Visual Axis in Hypermetropia

R, rest. The eyeball is of normal length and emmetropic. Hy, hypermetropia. The pull of the external and internal recti has been strengthened by advancement, and the retinoscope shows that hypermetropia has been produced. It may easily be noted that the eyeball is shorter. The rule shows that the focus of the camera was not appreciably changed between the taking of the two pictures.

Eyes from which the lens had been removed, or in which it had been pushed out of the axis of vision, responded to electrical stimulation precisely as did the normal eye, so long as the muscles were active; but when they had been paralyzed by the injection of atropine deep into the orbit, electrical stimulation had no effect on the refraction.

Fig. 20.   Lens Pushed Out of the Axis of Vision

In this experiment on the eye of a carp the lens was pushed out of the axis of vision. Accommodation took place after this displacement just as it did before. Note the point of the knife in the pupil in front of the lens.

In one experiment the lens was removed from the right eye of a rabbit, the refraction of each eye having first been tested by retinoscopy and found to be normal. The wound was then allowed to heal. Thereafter, for a period extending from one month to two years, electrical stimulation always produced accommodation in the lensless eye precisely to the same extent as in the eye which

Fig. 21.   Rabbit With Lens Removed

The animal was exhibited at a meeting of the Ophthalmological Section of the American Medical Association, held in Atlantic City, and was examined by a number of ophthalmologists present, all of whom testified that electrical stimulation of the eyeball produced accommodation, or myopic refraction, precisely as in the normal eye.

had a lens.   The same experiment with the same result was performed on a number of other rabbits, on dogs and on fish.   The obvious conclusion is that the lens is not a factor in accommodation.

In most text-books on physiology it is stated that accommodation is controlled by the third cranial nerve, which supplies all the muscles of the eyeball except the superior oblique and the external rectus; but the fourth cranial nerve, which supplies only the superior oblique, was found in these experiments to be just as much a nerve of accommodation as the third. When either the third or the fourth nerve was stimulated with electricity near its point of origin in the brain accommodation al-

Fig. 22. Experiment Upon the Eye of a Cat Demonstrating That the Fourth Nerve, Which Supplies Only the Superior Oblique Muscle, Is Just as Much a Nerve of Accommodation As the Third, and That the Superior Oblique Muscle Which It Supplies Is a Muscle of Accommodation.

No. 1.—Both nerves have been exposed near their origin in the brain, and a strip of black paper has been inserted beneath each to render it visible. The fourth nerve is the smaller one. The superior oblique muscle has been advanced by a tucking operation, as this muscle is always rudimentary in cats, and unless its pull is strengthened, accommodation cannot be produced in these animals. Stimulation of either or both nerves by the faradic current produced accommodation.

No. 2.—When the fourth nerve was covered with cotton soaked in a normal salt solution, the application of the faradic current to the cotton produced accommodation. When the cotton was soaked in a one per cent solution of atropine sulphate in a normal salt solution, such application produced no accommodation, but stimulation of the third nerve did produce it.

No. 3.—When the third nerve was covered with cotton soaked in a normal salt solution, the application of the faradic current to the cotton produced accommodation. When the cotton was soaked with atropine sulphate in a normal salt solution, such application produced no accommodation, but the stimulation of the fourth nerve did produce it.

No. 4.—When both nerves were covered with cotton soaked in atropine sulphate in a normal salt solution, the application of electricity to the cotton produced no accommodation. When the parts had been washed with a warm salt solution electrical stimulation of either nerve always produced accommodation. The nerves were alternately covered with the atropine-soaked cotton and then washed with the warm saline solution for an hour, the electricity being applied in each condition with invariably the same result. Accommodation could never be produced by electrical stimulation when the nerves were paralyzed with the atropine, but always resulted from the stimulation of either or both when they had been washed with the salt solution. The experiment was performed with the same results on many rabbits and dogs.

ways resulted in the normal eye. When the origin of either nerve was covered with a small wad of cotton soaked in a two per cent solution of atropine sulphate in a normal salt solution, stimulation of that nerve produced no accommodation, while stimulation of the unparalyzed nerve did produce it. When the origin of both nerves was covered with cotton soaked in atropine, accommodation could not be produced by electrical stimulation of either or both. When the cotton was removed and the nerves washed with normal salt solution, elec-

trical stimulation of either or both produced accommodation just as before the atropine had been applied. This
experiment, which was performed repeatedly for more

Fig. 23. Pithing a Fish Preparatory to Operating Upon
Its Eyes

The object of this operation is to secure greater relaxation of
the muscles of the eyes and head, which would work for hours,
without external stimulus, if the brain cells were not destroyed
by the probe.

than an hour by alternately applying and removing the
atropine, not only demonstrated clearly what had not
been known before, namely, that the fourth nerve is a
nerve of accommodation, but also demonstrated that the

superior oblique muscle which is supplied by it is an important factor in accommodation. It was further found that when the action of the oblique muscles was prevented by dividing them, the stimulation of the third nerve produced, not accommodation, but hypermetropia.

In all the experiments all sources of error are believed to have been eliminated. They were all repeated many times and always with the same result. They seemed, therefore, to leave no room for doubt that neither the lens nor any muscle inside the eyeball has anything to do with accommodation, but that the process whereby the eye adjusts itself for vision at different distances is entirely controlled by the action of the muscles on the outside of the globe.

CHAPTER V

THE TRUTH ABOUT ACCOMMODATION AS DEMON·STRATED BY A STUDY OF IMAGES REFLECTED FROM THE LENS, CORNEA, IRIS AND SCLERA

AS the conclusions in which the experiments described in the preceding chapter pointed were diametrically opposed to those reached by Helmholtz in his study of the images reflected from the front of the lens, I determined to repeat the experiments of the German investigator and find out, if possible, why his results were so different from my own. I devoted four years to this work, and was able to demonstrate that Helmholtz had erred through a defective technique, the image obtained by his method being so variable and uncertain that it lends itself to the support of almost any theory.

I worked for a year or more with the technique of Helmholtz, but was unable to obtain an image from the front of the lens which was sufficiently clear or distinct to be measured or photographed. With a naked candle as the source of light a clear and distinct image could be obtained on the cornea; on the back of the lens it was quite clear; but on the front of the lens it was very imperfect. Not only was it blurred, just as Helmholtz stated, but without any ascertainable cause it varied greatly in size and intensity. At times no reflection could be obtained at all, regardless of the angle of the light to the eye of the subject, or of the eye of the observer to that of the subject. With a diaphragm I got

Fig. 24.—Arrangements for Photographing Images Reflected
From the Eyeball

CM, concave mirror in which the subject may observe the
images reflected from various parts of her eye; C, condenser; D,
diaphragm; L, 1000-watt lamp; F, forehead rest; MP, bar which
the subject grasps with her teeth for the purpose of holding her
head steady; P, plane mirror upon which is pasted a letter of
diamond type and in which is reflected a Snellen test card twenty
feet behind the subject (the mirror is just above the letter P);
CAM, camera; Pr, perimeter used to measure the angle of the
light to the eye; R, plane mirror reflecting light from the 1000-
watt lamp upon the eye, which otherwise would be in total darkness except for the part from which the highly condensed image
of the filament is reflected; B, blue glass screen used to modify
the light reflected from the mirror R. When the subject read the
bottom line of the Snellen test card reflected in the mirror P,
her eye was at rest, and when she saw the letter of diamond type
distinctly it was accommodated ten diopters, as demonstrated by
the retinoscope.

Fig. 25. Arrangements for Holding the Head of the Subject
Steady While Images Were Being Photographed

CM, concave mirror; F, forehead rest; C, condenser, MP,
mouthpiece; Pr, perimeter.

a clearer and more constant image, but it still was not
sufficiently reliable to be measured. To Helmholtz the
indistinct image of a naked flame seemed to show an
appreciable change, while the images obtained by the
aid of the diaphragm showed it more clearly; but I was

unable, either with a diaphragm or without it, to obtain images which I considered sufficiently distinct to be reliable.

Men who had been teaching and demonstrating Helmholtz's theory repeated his experiments for my benefit; but the images which they obtained on the front of the lens did not seem to me any better than my own. After

Fig. 26. Image of Electric Filament on the Front of the Lens

R, rest; A, accommodation. Under the magnifying glass no change can be observed in the size of the two images. The image at the right looks larger only because it is more distinct. To support the theory of Helmholz it ought to be the smaller. The comet's tail at the left of the two images is an accidental reflection from the cornea. The spot of light beneath is a reflection from the light used to illuminate the eye while the photographs were being taken. It took two years to get these pictures.

studying these images almost daily for more than a year I was unable to make any reliable observation regarding the effect of accommodation upon them. In fact, it seemed that an infinite number of appearances might be obtained on the front of the lens when a candle was used as the source of illumination. At times the image became smaller during accommodation and seemed to sustain the theory of Helmholtz; but just as frequently it became larger. At other times it was impossible to tell what it did.

With a thirty-watt lamp, a fifty-watt lamp, a 250-watt lamp and a 1000-watt lamp, there was no improvement. The light of the sun reflected from the front of the lens produced an image just as cloudy and uncertain as the reflections from other sources of illumination, and just as variable in shape, intensity and size. To sum it all up, I was convinced that the anterior surface of the lens

Fig. 27. Images of the Electric Filament Reflected Simultaneously From the Cornea and Lens

R, rest; A, accommodation. The size of the images in both pictures is the same. The corneal image is so small that it has not been noticeably altered by the slight change that takes place in the cornea during accommodation. In A both images have changed their position and the end of the reflection from the lens has been cut off by the iris, but its width remains the same. The white spot between the two images of the filament is a reflection from the lamp used to illuminate the eye. Note that in A more of the sclera is visible, owing to the elongation of the eyeball during accommodation.

was a very poor reflector of light, and that no reliable images could be obtained from it by the means described.

After a year or more of failure I began to work at an aquarium on the eyes of fish. It was a long story of failure. Finally I became able, with the aid of a strong light—1000 watts—a diaphragm with a small opening and a condenser, to obtain, after some difficulty, a clear and distinct image from the cornea of fish. This image was sufficiently distinct to be measured, and after many months a satisfactory photograph was obtained. Then the work was resumed on the eyes of human beings. The strong light, combined with the diaphragm and condenser, the use of which was suggested by their use to improve the illumination of a glass slide under the microscope, proved to be a decided improvement over the method of Helmholtz, and by means of this technique an image was at last obtained on the front of the lens which was sufficiently clear and distinct to be photographed. This was the first time, so far as published records show, that an image of any kind was ever photographed from the front of the lens. Professional photographers whom I consulted with a view to securing their assistance assured me that the thing could not be done, and declined to attempt it. I was therefore obliged to learn photography, of which I have previously known nothing, myself, and I then found that so far as the image obtained by the method of Helmholtz is concerned the professionals were right.

The experiments were continued until, after almost four years of constant labor, I obtained satisfactory pictures before and after accommodation and during the production of myopia and hypermetropia, not only of images on the front of the lens, but of reflections from the iris, cornea, the front of the sclera (white of the eye) and the side of the sclera. I also became able to obtain images on any surface at will without reflections from the other parts. Before these results were obtained, however, many difficulties had still to be overcome.

Complicating reflections were a perpetual source of trouble. Reflections from surrounding objects were easily prevented; but those from the sides of the globe of the electric light were difficult to deal with, and it was useless to try to obtain images on the front of the lens until they had been eliminated, or reduced to a minimum, by

Fig. 28.   Image of Electric Filament Upon the Cornea

R, rest; A, accommodation. The image is smaller in A, but the change is so slight as to be scarcely noticeable, showing that the alteration in the shape of the cornea during accommodation is very slight.   For this reason the ophthalmometer, with its small image, has been thought to demonstrate that the cornea did not change during accommodation.

a proper adjustment of the light.   The same apparent adjustment did not, however, always give similar results. Sometimes there would be no reflections for days; then would come a day when, with the light apparently at the same angle, they would reappear.

With some adjustments of the light multiple images were seen reflected from the front of the lens. Sometimes these images were arranged in a horizontal line, sometimes in a vertical one and sometimes at angles of different degrees, while their distance from each other also varied. Usually there were three of them; some-times there were more; and sometimes there were only two. Occasionally they were all of the same size, but usually they varied, there being apparently no limit to their possibilities of change in this and other respects. Some of them were photographed, indicating that they were real reflections. Changes in the distance of the diaphragm from the light and from the condenser, and alterations in the size and shape of its opening, appeared to make no difference. Different adjustments of the con-denser were equally without effect. Changes in the angle at which the light was adjusted sometimes lessened the number of images and sometimes increased them, until at last an angle was found at which but one image was seen. The images appear, in fact, to have been caused by reflections from the globe of the electric light.

Even after the light had been so adjusted as to elimi-nate reflections it was often difficult, or impossible, to get a clear and distinct image of the electric filament upon the front of the lens. One could. rearrange the condenser and the diaphragm and change the axis of fixation, and still the image would be clouded or ob-scured and its outline distorted. The cause of the diffi-culty appeared to be that the light was not adjusted at the best angle for the purpose and it was not always possible to determine the exact axis at which a clear, distinct image would be produced. As in the case of the reflections from the sides of the globe, it seemed to vary without a known cause. This was true, however: that there were angles of the axis of the globe which gave better images than others, and that what these angles were could not be determined with exactness. I have

labored with the light for two or three hours without
finding the right angle. At other times the axis would
remain unchanged for days, giving always a clear, distinct image.

Fig. 29.   Image of Electric Filament on the Front of the Sclera

R, rest; A, accommodation.   During accommodation the front
of the sclera becomes more convex, because the eyeball has
elongated, just as a camera is elongated when it is focussed upon
a near object.   The spot of light on the cornea is an accidental
reflection.

The results of these experiments confirmed the conclusions drawn from the previous ones, namely, that accommodation is due to a lengthening of the eyeball, and not
to a change in the curvature of the lens.   They also confirmed, in a striking manner, my earlier conclusions as to
the conditions under which myopia and hypermetropia
are produced.[1]

The images photographed from the front of the lens
did not show any change in size or form during accommodation.   The image on the back of the lens also remained unchanged, as observed through the telescope
of the ophthalmometer; but as there is no dispute about
its behavior during accommodation, it was not photographed.   Images photographed from the iris before

[1] Bates: The Cause of Myopia, N. Y. Med. Jour., March 16, 1912.

and during accommodation were also the same in size and form, as was to be expected from the character of the lens images. If the lens changed during accommodation, the iris, which rests upon it, would change also.

Fig. 30. Images on the Side of the Sclera

R, rest; A, accommodation. The image in A is the larger, indicating a flattening of the side of the sclera as the eyeball elongates. My, Myopia. The eye is straining to see at the distance and the image is larger, indicating that the eyeball has elongated, resulting in a flattening of the side of the sclera. Hy, Hypermetropia. The eye is straining to see at two inches. The image is the smallest of the series, indicating that the eyeball has become shorter than in any of the other pictures, and the side of the sclera more convex. The two lower pictures confirm the author's previous observations that farsight is produced when the eye strains to see near objects and nearsight when it strains to see distant objects.

The images photographed from the cornea and from the front and side of the sclera showed, however, a series

Fig. 31. Multiple Images Upon the Front of the Lens

This picture illustrates one of the difficulties that had to be overcome in photographing images reflected from various parts of the eyeball. Unless the light was adjusted at precisely the right angle the filament was multiplied by reflection from the sides of the globe. Usually the image was doubled, sometimes it was tripled, as shown in the picture, and sometimes it was quadrupled. Often days of labor were required to eliminate these reflections, and for reasons that were not definitely determined the same adjustment did not always give the same results. Sometimes all would go well for days, and then, without any apparent reason, the multiple images would return.

of four well-marked changes, according to whether the vision was normal or accompanied by a strain. During accommodation the images from the cornea were smaller than when the eye was at rest, indicating elongation of the eyeball and a consequent increase in the convexity of the cornea. But when an unsuccessful effort was made to see at the near-point, the image became larger, indicating that the cornea had become less convex, a condition which one would expect when the optic axis was shortened, as in hypermetropia. When a strain was made to see at a distance the image was smaller than when the eye was at rest, again indicating elongation of the eyeball and increased convexity of the cornea.

The images photographed from the front of the sclera showed the same series of changes as the corneal images, but those obtained from the side of the sclera were found to have changed in exactly the opposite manner, being larger where the former were smaller and vice versa, a

Fig. 32. Reflection of the Electric Filament From the Iris

This picture is shown to illustrate the fact that it is possible to get a reflection from any reflecting surface of the eyeball without reflections from the other parts, although these may be exposed. This is done by changing the angle of the light to the eye. In No. 1 observations of the eye at the time the picture was taken demonstrated that the image was from the iris, not from the cornea, and the fact is also apparent in the picture. (Compare the image with the corneal reflection in Fig. 28.) In No. 2, where the image overlaps the margin of the pupil, the fact that the reflection is from the iris is manifest from the circumstance that only part of the filament is seen. If it were from the cornea, the whole of it would be reflected. Note in this picture that there is no reflection from the lens. The images on the iris did not change their size or shape during accommodation, demonstrating again that the lens, upon which the iris rests, does not change its shape when the eye adjusts itself for near vision.

difference which one would naturally expect from the fact that when the front of the sclera becomes more convex the sides must become flatter.

When an effort was made to see at a distance the image reflected from the side of the sclera was larger than the image obtained when the eye was at rest, indi·cating that this part of the sclera had become less convex or flatter, because of elongation of the eyeball. The image obtained during normal accommodation was also larger than when the eye was at rest, indicating again a flattening of the side of the sclera. The image obtained, however, when an effort was made to see near was much smaller than any of the other images, indicating that the sclera had become more convex at the side, a condition which one would expect when the eyeball was shortened, as in hypermetropia.

The most pronounced of the changes were noted in the images reflected from the front of the sclera. Those on the side of the sclera were less marked, and, owing to the difficulty of photographing a white image on a white background, could not always be readily seen on the photographs. They were always plainly apparent, however, to the observer, and still more so to the subject, who regarded them in a concave mirror. The alterations in the size of the corneal image were so slight that they did not show at all in the photographs, except when the image was large, a fact which explains why the ophthalmometer, with its small image, has been thought to show that the cornea did not change during accommodation. They were always apparent, however, to the subject and observer.

The corneal image was one of the easiest of the series to produce and the experiment is one which almost any-

Fig. 33. Demonstrating That the Back of the Lens Does Not Change During Accommodation

The filament of an electric light (L) is shining into the eye of the subject (S), and the reflection on the back of the lens can be seen by the observer (O) in the telescope (T). The subject holds in her hand, at a distance of four inches, a mirror on which is pasted a small letter, and in which is reflected a Snellen test card hung above and behind her head at a distance of twenty feet. The retinoscope reveals that when she looks at the reflection of the test card and reads the bottom line the eye is at rest, and that when she looks at the letter pasted on the mirror it accommodates. The image on the lens does not change during these changes of focus. The telescope is the telescope of the ophthalmometer, the prisms having been removed. As there is no dispute about the behavior of the back of the lens during accommodation this image was not photographed.

one can repeat, the only apparatus required being a fifty candlepower lamp—an ordinary electric globe—and a concave mirror fastened to a rod which moves back and forth in a groove so that the distance of the mirror from the eye can be altered at will. A plane mirror might also be used; but the concave glass is better, because it magnifies the image. The mirror should be so arranged that it reflects the image of the electric filament on the cornea, and so that the eye of the subject can see this reflection by looking straight ahead. The image in the mirror is used as the point of fixation, and the distance at which the eye focuses is altered by altering the distance of the mirror from the eye. The light can be placed within an inch or two of the eye, as the heat is not great enough to interfere with the experiment. The closer it is the larger the image, and according to whether it is adjusted vertically, horizontally, or at an angle, the clearness of the reflection may vary. A blue glass screen can be used, if desired, to lessen the discomfort of the light. If the left eye is used by the subject—and in all the experiments it was found to be the more convenient for the purpose—the source of light should be placed to the left of that eye and as much as possible to the front of it, at an angle of about forty-five degrees. For absolute accuracy the light and the head of the subject should be held immovable, but for demonstration this is not essential. Simply holding the bulb in his hand the subject can demonstrate that the image changes according to whether the eye is at rest, accommodating normally for near vision, or straining to see at a near or a distant point.

In the original report were described possible sources of error and the means taken to eliminate them.

CHAPTER VI

THE TRUTH ABOUT ACCOMMODATION AS DEMON-STRATED BY CLINICAL OBSERVATIONS

THE testimony of the experiments described in the preceding chapters to the effect that the lens is not a factor in accommodation is confirmed by numerous observations on the eyes of adults and children, with normal vision, errors of refraction, or amblyopia, and on the eyes of adults after the removal of the lens for cataract.

It has already been pointed out that the instillation of atropine into the eye is supposed to prevent accommodation by paralyzing the muscle credited with controlling the shape of the lens. That it has this effect is stated in every text-book on the subject,[1] and the drug is daily used in the fitting of glasses for the purpose of eliminating the supposed influence of the lens upon refractive states.

In about nine cases out of ten the conditions resulting from the instillation of atropine into the eye fit the theory upon which its use is based; but in the tenth case they do not, and every ophthalmologist of any experience has noted some of these tenth cases. Many of them are reported in the literature, and many of them have come under my own observation. According to the theory,

---

[1] Certain substances have the power of producing a dilation of the pupil (mydriasis), and hence are termed mydriatics. At the same time they act upon the ciliary body, diminishing and, when applied in sufficient strength, completely paralyzing the power of accommodation, thus rendering the eye for some time unalterably focussed for the farthest point.—Herman Snellen, Jr.: Mydriatics and Myotics, System of Diseases of the Eye, edited by Norris and Oliver, 1897-1900, vol. ii, p. 30.

atropine ought to bring out latent hypermetropia in eyes either apparently normal, or manifestly hypermetropic, provided, of course, the patient is of the age during which the lens is supposed to retain its elasticity. The fact is that it sometimes produces myopia, or changes hypermetropia into myopia, and that it will produce both myopia and hypermetropia in persons over seventy years of age, when the lens is supposed to be as hard as a stone, as well as in cases in which the lens is hard with incipient cataract. Patients with eyes apparently normal will, after the use of atropine, develop hypermetropic astigmatism, or myopic astigmatism, or compound myopic astigmatism, or mixed astigmatism.[1] In other cases the drug will not interfere with the accommodation, or alter the refraction in any way. Furthermore, when the vision has been lowered by atropine the subjects have often become able, simply by resting their eyes, to read diamond type at six inches. Yet atropine is supposed to rest the eyes by affording relief to an overworked muscle.

In the treatment of squint and amblyopia I have often used atropine in the better eye for more than a year, in order to encourage the use of the amblyopic eye; and at the end of this time, while still under the influence of atropine, such eyes have become able in a few hours, or less, to read diamond type at six inches (see Chapter XXII). The following are examples of many similar cases that might be cited:

A boy of ten had hypermetropia in both eyes, that of

---

[1] In simple hypermetropic astigmatism one principal meridian is normal and the other, at right angles to it, is flatter. In simple myopic astigmatism the contrary is the case; one principal meridian is normal and the other, at right angles to it, more convex. In mixed astigmatism one principal meridian is too flat, the other too convex. In compound hypermetropic astigmatism both principal meridians are flatter than normal, one more so than the other. In compound myopic astigmatism both are more convex than normal, one more so than the other.

the left or better eye amounting to three diopters. When atropine was instilled into this eye the hypermetropia was increased to four and a half diopters, and the vision lowered to 20/200. With a convex glass of four and a half diopters the patient obtained normal vision for the distance, and with the addition of another convex glass of four diopters he was able to read diamond type at ten inches (best). The atropine was used for a year, the pupil being dilated continually to the maximum. Meantime the right eye was being treated by methods to be described later. Usually in such cases the eye which is not being specifically treated improves to some extent with the others, but in this case it did not. At the end of the year the vision of the right eye had become normal; but that of the left eye remained precisely what it was at the beginning, being still 20/200 without glasses for the distance, while reading without glasses was impossible and the degree of the hypermetropia had not changed. Still under the influence of the atropine and still with the pupil dilated to the maximum, this eye was now treated separately; and in half an hour its vision had become normal both for the distance and the nearpoint, diamond type being read at six inches, all without glasses. According to the accepted theories, the ciliary muscle of this eye must not only have been completely paralyzed at the time, but must have been in a state of complete paralysis for a year. Yet the eye not only overcame four and a half diopters of hypermetropia, but added six diopters of accommodation, making a total of ten and a half. It remains for those who adhere to the accepted theories to say how such facts can be reconciled with them.

Equally, if not more remarkable, was the case of a

little girl of six who had two and a half diopters of hypermetropia in her right or better eye, and six in the other, with one diopter of astigmatism. With the better eye under the influence of atropine and the pupil dilated to the maximum, both eyes were treated together for more than a year, and at the end of that time, the right being still under the influence of the atropine, both became able to read diamond type at six inches, the right doing it better, if anything, than the left. Thus, in spite of the atropine, the right eye not only overcame two and a half diopters of hypermetropia, but added six diopters of accommodation, making a total of eight and a half. In order to eliminate all possibility of latent hypermetropia in the left eye—which in the beginning had six diopters —the atropine was now used in this eye and discontinued in the other, the eye education being continued as before. Under the influence of the drug there was a slight return of the hypermetropia; but the vision quickly became normal again, and although the atropine was used daily for more than a year, the pupil being continually dilated to the maximum, it remained so, diamond type being read at six inches without glasses during the whole period. It is difficult for me to conceive how the ciliary muscle could have had anything to do with the ability of this patient to accommodate after atropine had been used in each eye separately for a year or more at a time.

According to the current theory, atropine paralyzes the ciliary muscle and thus, by preventing a change of curvature in the lens, prevents accommodation. When accommodation occurs, therefore, after the prolonged use of atropine, it is evident that it must be due to some factor or factors other than the lens and the ciliary muscle. The evidence of such cases against the accepted theories is, in fact, overwhelming; and according to these theories the other factors cited in this chapter are equally inexplicable. All of these facts, however, are in entire accord with the results of my experiments on the eye muscles of animals and my observations regarding the behavior of images reflected from various parts of the eyeball. They strikingly confirm, too, the testimony of the experiments with atropine, which showed that the accommodation could not be paralyzed completely and permanently unless the atropine was injected deep into the orbit, so as to reach the oblique muscles, the real muscles of accommodation, while hypermetropia could not be prevented when the eyeball was stimulated with electricity without a similar use of atropine, resulting in the paralysis of the recti muscles.

As has already been noted, the fact that after the removal of the lens for cataract the eye often appears to accommodate just as well as it did before is well known. Many of these cases have come under my own observation. Such patients have not only read diamond type with only their distance glasses on, at thirteen and ten inches and at a less distance, but one man was able to read without any glass at all. In all these cases the retinoscope demonstrated that the apparent act of accommodation was real, being accomplished, not by the "interpretation of circles of diffusion," or by any of the other methods by which this inconvenient phenomenon is commonly explained, but by an accurate adjustment of the focus to the distances concerned.

The cure of presbyopia (see Chapter XX) must also be added to the clinical testimony against the accepted theory of accommodation. On the theory that the lens is a factor in accommodation such cures would be manifestly impossible. The fact that rest of the eyes improves the sight in presbyopia has been noted by others, and has been attributed to the supposed fact that the rested ciliary muscle is able for a brief period to influence the hardened lens; but while it is conceivable that this might happen in the early stages of the condition and for a few moments, it is not conceivable that permanent relief should be obtained by this means, or that lenses which are, as the saying goes, as "hard as a stone," should be influenced, even momentarily.

A truth is strengthened by an accumulation of facts. A working hypothesis is proved not to be a truth if a single fact is not in harmony with it. The accepted theories of accommodation and of the cause of errors of refraction require that a multitude of facts shall be explained away. During more than thirty years of clinical experience, I have not observed a single fact that was not in harmony with the belief that the lens and the ciliary muscle have nothing to do with accommodation, and that the changes in the shape of the eyeball upon which errors of refraction depend are not permanent. My clinical observations have of themselves been sufficient to demonstrate this fact. They have also been sufficient to show how errors of refraction can be produced at will, and how they may be cured, temporarily in a few minutes, and permanently by continued treatment.

CHAPTER VII

THE VARIABILITY OF THE REFRACTION OF
THE EYE

THE theory that errors of refraction are due to permanent deformations of the eyeball leads naturally to the conclusion, not only that errors of refraction are permanent states, but that normal refraction is also a continuous condition. As this theory is almost universally accepted as a fact, therefore, it is not surprising to find that the normal eye is generally regarded as a perfect machine which is always in good working order. No matter whether the object regarded is strange or familiar, whether the light is good or imperfect, whether the surroundings are pleasant or disagreeable, even under conditions of nerve strain or bodily disease, the normal eye is expected to have normal refraction and normal sight all the time. It is true that the facts do not harmonize with this view, but they are conveniently attributed to the perversity of the ciliary muscle, or if that explanation will not work, ignored altogether.

When we understand, however, how the shape of the eyeball is controlled by the external muscles, and how it responds instantaneously to their action, it is easy to see that no refractive state, whether it is normal or abnormal, can be permanent. This conclusion is confirmed by the retinoscope, and I had observed the facts long before the experiments described in the preceding chapters had offered a satisfactory explanation for it. During thirty years devoted to the study of refraction, I have found few people who could maintain perfect sight for more than a few minutes at a time, even under the most favorable conditions; and often I have seen the refraction change half a dozen times or more in a second, the variations ranging all the way from twenty diopters of myopia to normal.

Similarly I have found no eyes with continuous or unchanging errors of refraction, all persons with errors of refraction having, at frequent intervals during the day and night, moments of normal vision, when their myopia, hypermetropia, or astigmatism, wholly disappears.   The form of the error also changes, myopia even changing into hypermetropia, and one form of astigmatism into another.

Of twenty thousand school children examined in one year, more than half had normal eyes, with sight which was perfect at times; but not one of them had perfect sight in each eye at all times of the day.   Their sight might be good in the morning and imperfect in the afternoon, or imperfect in the morning and perfect in the afternoon.   Many children could read one Snellen test card with perfect sight, while unable to see a different one perfectly.   Many could also read some letters of the alphabet perfectly, while unable to distinguish other letters of the same size under similar conditions.   The degree of this imperfect sight varied within wide limits, from one-third to one-tenth, or less.   Its duration was also variable.   Under some conditions it might continue for only a few minutes, or less; under others it might prevent the subject from seeing the blackboard for days, weeks, or even longer.   Frequently all the pupils in a classroom were affected to this extent.

Among babies a similar condition was noted.   Most

investigators have found babies hypermetropic. A few have found them myopic. My own observations indicate that the refraction of infants is continually changing. One child was examined under atropine on four successive days, beginning two hours after birth. A three per cent solution of atropine was instilled into both eyes, the pupil was dilated to the maximum, and other physiological symptoms of the use of atropine were noted. The first examination showed a condition of mixed astigmatism. On the second day there was compound hypermetropic astigmatism, and on the third compound myopic astigmatism. On the fourth one eye was normal and the other showed simple myopia. Similar variations were noted in many other cases.

What is true of children and infants is equally true of adults of all ages. Persons over seventy years of age have suffered losses of vision of variable degree and intensity, and in such cases the retinoscope always indicated an error of refraction. A man eighty years old, with normal eyes and ordinarily normal sight, had periods of imperfect sight which would last from a few minutes to half an hour or longer. Retinoscopy at such times always indicated myopia of four diopters or more.

During sleep the refractive condition of the eye is rarely, if ever, normal. Persons whose refraction is normal when they are awake will produce myopia, hypermetropia and astigmatism when they are asleep, or, if they have errors of refraction when they are awake, they will be increased during sleep. This is why people waken in the morning with eyes more tired than at any other time, or even with severe headaches. When the subject is under ether or chloroform, or unconscious from any other cause, errors of refraction are also produced or increased.

When the eye regards an unfamiliar object an error of refraction is always produced. Hence the proverbial fatigue caused by viewing pictures, or other objects, in a museum. Children with normal eyes who can read perfectly small letters a quarter of an inch high at ten feet always have trouble in reading strange writing on the blackboard, athough the letters may be two inches high. A strange map, or any map, has the same effect. I have never seen a child, or a teacher, who could look at a map at the distance without becoming nearsighted. German type has been accused of being responsible for much of the poor sight once supposed to be peculiarly a German malady; but if a German child attempts to read Roman print, it will at once become temporarily hypermetropic. German print, or Greek or Chinese characters, will have the same effect on a child, or other person, accustomed to Roman letters. Cohn repudiated the idea that German lettering was trying to the eyes.[1] On the contrary, he always found it "pleasant, after a long reading of the monotonous Roman print, to return 'to our beloved German.'" Because the German characters were more familiar to him than any others he found them restful to his eyes. "Use," as he truly observed, "has much to do with the matter." Children learning to read, write, draw, or sew, always suffer from defective vision, because of the unfamiliarity of the lines or objects with which they are working.

A sudden exposure to strong light, or rapid or sudden changes of light, are likely to produce imperfect sight in the normal eye, continuing in some cases for weeks and months (see Chapter XVII).

---

[1] Eyes and School Books, Pop. Sci. Monthly, May, 1881, translated from Deutsche Rundschau.

Noise is also a frequent cause of defective vision in the normal eye. All persons see imperfectly when they hear an unexpected loud noise. Familiar sounds do not lower the vision, but unfamiliar ones always do. Country children from quiet schools may suffer from defective vision for a long time after moving to a noisy city. In school they cannot do well with their work, because their sight is impaired. It is, of course, a gross injustice for teachers and others to scold, punish, or humiliate such children.

Under conditions of mental or physical discomfort, such as pain, cough, fever, discomfort from heat or cold, depression, anger, or anxiety, errors of refraction are always produced in the normal eye, or increased in the eye in which they already exist.

The variability of the refraction of the eye is responsible for many otherwise unaccountable accidents. When people are struck down in the street by automobiles, or trolley cars, it is often due to the fact that they were suffering from temporary loss of sight. Collisions on railroads or at sea, disasters in military operations, aviation accidents, etc., often occur because some responsible person suffered temporary loss of sight.

To this cause must also be ascribed, in a large degree, the confusion which every student of the subject has noted in the statistics which have been collected regarding the occurrence of errors of refraction. So far as I am aware it has never been taken into account by any investigator of the subject; yet the result in any such investigation must be largely determined by the conditions under which it is made. It is possible to take the best eyes in the world and test them so that the subject will not be able to get into the Army. Again, the test may be so made that eyes which are apparently much below normal at the beginning, may in the few minutes required for the test, acquire normal vision and become able to read the test card perfectly.

CHAPTER VIII

WHAT GLASSES DO TO US

THE Florentines were doubtless mistaken in supposing that their fellow citizen (see page v) was the inventor of the lenses now so commonly worn to correct errors of refraction. There has been much discussion as to the origin of these devices, but they are generally believed to have been known at a period much earlier than that of Salvino degli Armati. The Romans at least must have known something of the art of supplementing the powers of the eye, for Pliny tells us that Nero used to watch the games in the Colosseum through a concave gem set in a ring for that purpose. If, however, his contemporaries believed that Salvino of the Armati was the first to produce these aids to vision, they might well pray for the pardon of his sins; for while it is true that eyeglasses have brought to some people improved vision and relief from pain and discomfort, they have been to others simply an added torture, they always do more or less harm, and at their best they never improve the vision to normal.

That glasses cannot improve the sight to normal can be very simply demonstrated by looking at any color through a strong convex or concave glass. It will be noted that the color is always less intense than when seen with the naked eye; and since the perception of form depends upon the perception of color, it follows that both color and form must be less distinctly seen with glasses than without them. Even plane glass lowers the vision both for color and form, as everyone knows who has ever looked out of a window. Women who wear glasses for minor defects of vision often observe that they are made more or less color-blind by them, and in a shop one may note that they remove them when they want to match samples. If the sight is seriously defective, the color may be seen better with glasses than without them.

That glasses must injure the eye is evident from the facts given in the preceding chapter. One cannot see through them unless one produces the degree of refractive error which they are designed to correct. But refractive errors, in the eye which is left to itself, are never constant. If one secures good vision by the aid of concave, or convex, or astigmatic lenses, therefore, it means that one is maintaining constantly a degree of refractive error which otherwise would not be maintained constantly. It is only to be expected that this should make the condition worse, and it is a matter of common experience that it does. After people once begin to wear glasses their strength, in most cases, has to be steadily increased in order to maintain the degree of visual acuity secured by the aid of the first pair. Persons with presbyopia who put on glasses because they cannot read fine print too often find that after they have worn them for a time they cannot, without their aid, read the larger print that was perfectly plain to them before. A person with myopia of 20/70 who puts on glasses giving him a vision of 20/20 may find that in a week's time his unaided vision has declined to 20/200, and we have the testimony of Dr. Sidler-Huguenin, of Zurich,[1] that of the thousands of myopes treated by him the majority grew steadily worse, in spite of all the skill he could apply to the fitting of glasses for them. When people break their glasses and go without them for a week or two, they

---

[1] Archiv. f. Augenh., vol. lxxix, 1915, translated in Arch. Ophth., vol. xlv, Nov. 6, 1916.

frequently observe that their sight has improved. As a matter of fact the sight always improves, to a greater or less degree, when glasses are discarded, although the fact may not always be noted.

That the human eye resents glasses is a fact which no one would attempt to deny. Every oculist knows that patients have to "get used" to them, and that sometimes they never succeed in doing so. Patients with high degrees of myopia and hypermetropia have great difficulty in accustoming themselves to the full correction, and often are never able to do so. The strong concave glasses required by myopes of high degree make all objects seem much smaller than they really are, while convex glasses enlarge them. These are unpleasantnesses that cannot be overcome. Patients with high degrees of astigmatism suffer some very disagreeable sensations when they first put on glasses, for which reason they are warned by one of the "Conservation of Vision" leaflets published by the Council on Health and Public Instruction of the American Medical Association to "get used to them at home before venturing where a misstep might cause a serious accident."[1] Usually these difficulties are overcome, but often they are not, and it sometimes happens that those who get on fairly well with their glasses in the daytime never succeed in getting used to them at night.

All glasses contract the field of vision to a greater or less degree. Even with very weak glasses patients are unable to see distinctly unless they look through the center of the lenses, with the frames at right angles to the line of vision; and not only is their vision lowered if they fail to do this, but annoying nervous symptoms,

---

[1] Lancaster: Wearing Glasses, p. 15.

such as dizziness and headache, are sometimes produced. Therefore they are unable to turn their eyes freely in different directions. It is true that glasses are now ground in such a way that it is theoretically possible to look through them at any angle, but practically they seldom accomplish the desired result.

The difficulty of keeping the glass clear is one of the minor discomforts of glasses, but nevertheless a most annoying one. On damp and rainy days the atmosphere clouds them. On hot days the perspiration from the body may have a similar effect. On cold days they are often clouded by the moisture of the breath. Every day they are so subject to contamination by dust and moisture and the touch of the fingers incident to unavoidable handling that it is seldom they afford an absolutely unobstructed view of the objects regarded.

Reflections of strong light from eyeglasses are often very annoying, and in the street may be very dangerous.

Soldiers, sailors, athletes, workmen and children have great difficulty with glasses because of the activity of their lives, which not only leads to the breaking of the lenses, but often throws them out of focus, particularly in the case of eyeglasses worn for astigmatism.

The fact that glasses are very disfiguring may seem a matter unworthy of consideration in a medical publication; but mental discomfort does not improve either the general health or the vision, and while we have gone so far toward making a virtue of what we conceive to be necessity that some of us have actually come to consider glasses becoming, huge round lenses in ugly tortoise-shell frames being positively fashionable at the present time, there are still some unperverted minds to which the wearing of glasses is mental torture and the sight of them upon others far from agreeable. Most human beings are, unfortunately, ugly enough without putting glasses upon them, and to disfigure any of the really beautiful faces that we have with such contrivances is surely as bad as putting an import tax upon art. As for putting glasses upon a child it is enough to make the angels weep.

Up to a generation ago glasses were used only as an aid to defective sight, but they are now prescribed for large numbers of persons who can see as well or better without them. As explained in Chapter I, the hypermetropic eye is believed to be capable of correcting its own difficulties to some extent by altering the curvature of the lens, through the activity of the ciliary muscle. The eye with simple myopia is not credited with this capacity, because an increase in the convexity of the lens, which is supposed to be all that is accomplished by accommodative effort, would only increase the difficulty; but myopia is usually accompanied by astigmatism, and this, it is believed, can be overcome, in part, by alterations in the curvature of the lens. Thus we are led by the theory to the conclusion that an eye in which any error of refraction exists is practically never free, while open, from abnormal accommodative efforts. In other words, it is assumed that the supposed muscle of accommodation has to bear, not only the normal burden of changing the focus of the eye for vision at different distances, but the additional burden of compensating for refractive errors. Such adjustments, if they actually took place, would naturally impose a severe strain upon the nervous system, and it is to relieve this strain—which is believed to be the cause of a host of functional nervous troubles— quite as much as to improve the sight, that glasses are prescribed.

It has been demonstrated, however, that the lens is not

a factor, either in the production of accommodation, or in the correction of errors of refraction. Therefore under no circumstances can there be a strain of the ciliary muscle to be relieved. It has also been demonstrated that when the vision is normal no error of refraction is present, and the extrinsic muscles of the eyeball are at rest. Therefore there can be no strain of the extrinsic muscles to be relieved in these cases. When a strain of these muscles does exist, glasses may correct its effects upon the refraction, but the strain itself they cannot relieve. On the contrary, as has been shown, they must make it worse. Nevertheless persons with normal vision who wear glasses for the relief of a supposed muscular strain are often benefited by them. This is a striking illustration of the effect of mental suggestion, and plane glass, if it could inspire the same faith, would produce the same result. In fact, many patients have told me that they had been relieved of various discomforts by glasses which I found to be simply plane glass. One of these patients was an optician who had fitted the glasses himself and was under no illusions whatever about them; yet he assured me that when he didn't wear them he got headaches.

Some patients are so responsive to mental suggestion that you can relieve their discomfort, or improve their sight, with almost any glasses you like to put on them. I have seen people with hypermetropia wearing myopic glasses with a great deal of comfort, and people with no astigmatism getting much satisfaction from glasses designed for the correction of this defect.

Landolt mentions the case of a patient who had for years worn prisms for insufficiency of the internal recti, and who found them absolutely indispensable for work, although the apices were toward the nose. The prescription, which the patient was able to produce, called for prisms adjusted in the usual manner, with the apices toward the temples; but the optician had made a mistake which, owing to the patient's satisfaction with the result, had never been discovered. Landolt explained the case by "the slight effect of weak prisms and the great power of imagination";[1] and doubtless the benefit derived from the glasses was real, resulting from the patient's great faith in the specialist—described as "one of the most competent of ophthalmologists"—who prescribed them.

Some patients will even imagine that they see better with glasses that markedly lower the vision. A number of years ago a patient for whom I had prescribed glasses consulted an ophthalmologist whose reputation was much greater than my own, and who gave him another pair of glasses and spoke slightingly of the ones that I had prescribed. The patient returned to me and told me how much better he could see with the second pair of glasses than he did with the first. I tested his vision with the new glasses, and found that while mine had given him a vision of 20/20 those of my colleague enabled him to see only 20/40. The simple fact was that he had been hypnotized by a great reputation into thinking he could see better when he actually saw worse; and it was hard to convince him that he was wrong, although he had to admit that when he looked at the test card he could see only half as much with the new glasses as with the old ones.

When glasses do not relieve headaches and other nervous symptoms it is assumed to be because they were not properly fitted, and some practitioners and their patients exhibit an astounding degree of patience and

---

[1] Anomalies of the Motor Apparatus of the Eye, System of Diseases of the Eye, vol. iv, pp. 154-155.

perseverance in their joint attempts to arrive at the proper prescription. A patient who suffered from severe pains at the base of his brain was fitted sixty times by one specialist alone, and had besides visited many other eye and nerve specialists in this country and in Europe. He was relieved of the pain in five minutes by the methods presented in this book, while his vision, at the same time, became temporarily normal.

It is fortunate that many people for whom glasses have been prescribed refuse to wear them, thus escaping not only much discomfort but much injury to their eyes. Others, having less independence of mind, or a larger share of the martyr's spirit, or having been more badly frightened by the oculists, submit to an amount of unnecessary torture which is scarcely conceivable. One such patient wore glasses for twenty-five years, although they did not prevent her from suffering continual misery and lowered her vision to such an extent that she had to look over the tops when she wanted to see anything at a distance. Her oculist assured her that she might expect the most serious consequences if she did not wear the glasses, and was very severe about her practice of looking over instead of through them.

As refractive abnormalities are continually changing, not only from day to day and from hour to hour, but from minute to minute, even under the influence of atropine, the accurate fitting of glasses is, of course, impossible. In some cases these fluctuations are so extreme, or the patient so unresponsive to mental suggestion, that no relief whatever is obtained from correcting lenses, which necessarily become under such circumstances an added discomfort. At their best it cannot be maintained that glasses are anything more than a very unsatisfactory substitute for normal vision.

CHAPTER IX

THE CAUSE AND CURE OF ERRORS OF REFRACTION

IT has been demonstrated in thousands of cases that all abnormal action of the external muscles of the eyeball is accompanied by a strain or effort to see, and that with the relief of this strain the action of the muscles becomes normal and all errors of refraction disappear. The eye may be blind, it may be suffering from atrophy of the optic nerve, from cataract, or disease of the retina; but so long as it does not try to see, the external muscles act normally and there is no error of refraction. This fact furnishes us with the means by which all these conditions, so long held to be incurable, may be cured.

It has also been demonstrated that for every error of refraction there is a different kind of strain. The study of images reflected from various parts of the eyeball confirmed what had previously been observed, namely, that myopia (or a lessening of hypermetropia) is always associated with a strain to see at the distance, while hypermetropia (or a lessening of myopia) is always associated with a strain to see at the near-point; and the fact can be verified in a few minutes by anyone who knows how to use a retinoscope, provided only that the instrument is not brought nearer to the subject than six feet.

In an eye with previously normal vision a strain to see near objects always results in the temporary production of hypermetropia in one or all meridians. That is, the eye either becomes entirely hypermetropic, or some form

89

Patient reading fine print in a good light at thirteen inches, the object of vision being placed above the eye so as to be out of the line of the camera. Simultaneous retinoscopy indicated that the eye was focused at thirteen inches. The glass was used with the retinoscope to determine the amount of the refraction.

Fig. 34.   Straining to See at the Near-Point Produces Hypermetropia

When the room was darkened the patient failed to read the fine print at thirteen inches and the retinoscope indicated that the eye was focused at a greater distance. When a conscious strain of considerable degree was made to see, the eye became hypermetropic.

Fig. 35 Myopia Produced by unconscious Strain to See at the Distance is Increased by Conscious Strain.

No. 1.—Normal vision.

No. 2.—Same subject four years later with myopia. Note the strained expression.

No. 3.—Myopia increased by conscious effort to see a distant object.

Fig. 36. Immediate Production of Myopia and Myopic Astigmatism in Eyes Previously Normal by Strain to See at the Distance

Boy reading the Snellen test card with normal vision. Note the absence of facial strain.

The same boy trying to see a picture at twenty feet. The effort, manifested by staring, produces compound myopic astigmatism, as revealed by the retinoscope.

of astigmatism is produced of which hypermetropia forms a part. In the hypermetropic eye the hypermetropia is increased in one or all meridians. When the myopic eye strains to see a near object the myopia is lessened and emmetropia[1] may be produced, the eye being focussed for parallel rays while still trying to see at the near-point. In some cases the emmetropia may even pass over into hypermetropia in one or all meridians. All these changes are accompanied by evidences of increasing strain, in the form of eccentric fixation (see Chapter XI) and lowered vision; but, strange to say, pain and fatigue are usually relieved to a marked degree. If, on the contrary, the eye with previously normal vision strains to see at the distance, temporary myopia is always produced in one or all meridians, and if the eye is already myopic, the myopia is increased. If the hypermetropic eye strains to see a distant object, pain and fatigue may be produced or increased; but the hypermetropia and the eccen-

The same boy making himself myopic voluntarily by partly closing the eyelids and making a conscious effort to read the test card at ten feet.

[1] Emmetropia (from the Greek *emmetros*, in measure, and *ops*, the eye) is that condition of the eye in which it is focussed for parallel rays. This constitutes normal vision at the distance, but is an error of refraction when it occurs at the near-point.

tric fixation are lessened and the vision improves. This interesting result, it will be noted, is the exact contrary of what we get when the myope strains to see at the near-point. In some cases the hypermetropia is completely relieved, and emmetropia is produced, with a complete disappearance of all evidences of strain. This condition may then pass over into myopia, with an increase of strain as the myopia increases.

In other words the eye which strains to see at the near-point becomes flatter than it was before, in one or all meridians. If it was elongated to start with, it may pass

Fig. 37. Myopic Astigmatism comes and Goes According as the Subject Looks at Distant Objects With or Without Strain

No. 1.—Patient regarding the Snellen test card at ten feet without effort and reading the bottom line with normal vision.

No. 2.—The same patient making an effort to see a picture at twenty feet. The retinoscope indicated compound myopic astigmatism.

from this condition through emmetropia, in which it is spherical, to hypermetropia, in which it is flattened; and if these changes take place unsymmetrically, astigmatism will be produced in connection with the other conditions. The eye which strains to see at the distance, on the contrary, becomes longer than it was before in one or all meridians, and may pass from the flattened condition of hypermetropia, through emmetropia, to the elongated condition of myopia. If these changes take place unsymmetrically, astigmatism will again be produced in connection with the other conditions.

What has been said of the normal eye applies equally to eyes from which the lens has been removed. This operation produces usually a condition of hypermetropia; but when there has previously been a condition of high myopia the removal of the lens may not be sufficient to correct it, and the eye may still remain myopic. In the first case a strain to see at the distance lessens the hypermetropia, and a strain to see at the near-point increases it; in the second a strain to see at the distance increases the myopia, and a strain to see at the near-point lessens it. For a longer or shorter period after the removal of the lens many aphakic eyes strain to see at the near-point, producing so much hypermetropia that the patient cannot read ordinary print, and the power of accommodation appears to have been completely lost. Later, when the patient becomes accustomed to the situation, this strain is often relieved, and the eye becomes able to focus accurately upon near objects. Some rare cases have also been observed in which a measure of good vision both for distance and the near-point was obtained without glasses, the eyeball elongating sufficiently to compensate, to some degree, for the loss of the lens.

Fig. 38.   This Patient Had Had the Lens of the Right Eye Removed for Cataract and Was Wearing an Artificial Eye in the Left Socket.   The Removal of the Lens created a Condition of Hypermetropia Which Was Corrected by a Convex Glass of Ten Diopters.

No. 1.—The patient is reading the Snellen test card at twenty feet with normal vision. No. 2.—She is straining to see the test card at the same distance, and her hypermetropia is lessened by two diopters so that her glass now overcorrects it and she cannot see the card perfectly. No. 3.—With a convex reading glass of thirteen diopters the right eye is focussed accurately at thirteen inches. No. 4.—The patient is straining to see at the same distance and her hypermetropia is so increased that in order to read she would require a glass of fifteen diopters. On the basis of the accepted theory that the power of accommodation is wholly destroyed by the removal of the lens these changes in the refraction would have been impossible. The experiment was repeated several times and it was found that the error of refraction produced by straining to see varied, being sometimes more and sometimes less than two diopters.

The phenomena associated with strain in the human eye have also been observed in the eyes of the lower animals. I have made many dogs myopic by inducing them to strain to see a distant object. One very nervous dog, with normal refraction, as demonstrated by the retinoscope, was allowed to smell a piece of meat. He became very much excited, pricked up his ears, arched his eyebrows and wagged his tail. The meat was then removed to a distance of twenty feet. The dog looked disappointed, but didn't lose interest. While he was watching the meat it was dropped into a box. A worried look came into his eyes. He strained to see what had become of it, and the retinoscope showed that he had become myopic. This experiment, it should be added, would succeed only with an animal possessing two active oblique muscles. Animals in which one of these muscles is absent or rudimentary are unable to elongate the eyeball under any circumstances.

Primarily the strain to see is a strain of the mind, and, as in all cases in which there is a strain of the mind, there is a loss of mental control. Anatomically the results of straining to see at a distance may be the same as those of regarding an object at the near point without strain; but in one case the eye does what the mind desires; and in the other it does not.

These facts appear sufficiently to explain why visual acuity declines as civilization advances. Under the conditions of civilized life men's minds are under a continual strain. They have more things to worry them than uncivilized man had, and they are not obliged to keep cool and collected in order that they may see and do other things upon which existence depends. If he allowed himself to get nervous, primitive man was promptly eliminated; but civilized man survives and transmits his mental characteristics to posterity. The lower animals when subjected to civilized conditions respond to them in precisely the same way as do human creatures. I have examined many domestic and menagerie animals, and have found them, in many cases, myopic, although they neither read, nor write, nor sew, nor set type.

A decline in visual acuity at the distance, however, is

Fig. 39.   A Family Group Strikingly Illustrating the Effect of the Mind Upon the Vision

No. 1.—Girl of four with normal eyes.   No. 2.—The child's mother with myopia.   No. 3—The same girl at nine with myopia. Note that her expression has completely changed, and is now exactly like her mother's.   Nos. 4, 5 and 6.—The girl's brother at two, six and eight.   His eyes are normal in all three pictures. The girl has either inherited her mother's disposition to take things hard, or has been injuriously effected by her personality of strain.   The boy has escaped both influences.   In view of the prevailing theories about the relation of heredity to myopia, this picture is particularly interesting.

no more a peculiarity of civilization than is a similar decline at the near-point. Myopes, although they see better at the near-point than they do at the distance, never see as well as does the eye with normal sight;

Fig. 40.   Myopes Who Never Went to School, or Read in the Subway

No. 1.—Myopic elephant in the Central Park Zoo, New York, thirty-nine years old. Young elephants and other young animals were found to have normal vision.

No. 2.—Cape buffalo with myopia, Central Park Zoo.

No. 3.—Myopic monkey, also in the Central Park Zoo.

No. 4.—Pet dog with myopia which progressed from year to year.

and in hypermetropia, which is more common than myopia, the sight is worse at the near-point than at the distance.

The remedy is not to avoid either near work or distant vision, but to get rid of the mental strain which underlies the imperfect functioning of the eye at both points; and it has been demonstrated in thousands of cases that this can always be done.

Fortunately, all persons are able to relax under certain conditions at will. In all uncomplicated errors of refraction the strain to see can be relieved, temporarily, by having the patient look at a blank wall without trying to see. To secure permanent relaxation sometimes requires considerable time and much ingenuity. The same method cannot be used with everyone. The ways in which people strain to see are infinite, and the methods used to relieve the strain must be almost equally varied. Whatever the method that brings most relief, however, the end is always the same, namely relaxation. By constant repetition and frequent demonstration and by all means possible, the fact must be impressed upon the patient that perfect sight can be obtained only by relaxation. Nothing else matters.

Most people, when told that rest, or relaxation, will cure their eye troubles, ask why sleep does not do so. The answer to this question was given in Chapter VII. The eyes are rarely, if ever, completely relaxed in sleep, and if they are under a strain when the subject is awake, that strain will certainly be continued during sleep, to a greater or less degree, just as a strain of other parts of the body is continued.

The idea that it rests the eyes not to use them is also erroneous. The eyes were made to see with, and if when they are open they do not see, it is because they are under such a strain and have such a great error of refraction that they cannot see. Near vision, although accomplished by a muscular act, is no more a strain on them than is distant vision, although accomplished without the intervention of the muscles. The use of the muscles does not necessarily produce fatigue. Some men can run for hours without becoming tired. Many birds support themselves upon one foot during sleep, the toes tightly clasping the swaying bough and the muscles remaining unfatigued by the apparent strain. Fabre tells of an insect which hung back downward for ten months from the roof of its wire cage, and in that position performed all the functions of life, even to mating and laying its eggs. Those who fear the effect of civilization, with its numerous demands for near vision, upon the eye may take courage from the example of this marvelous little animal which, in a state of nature, hangs by its feet only at intervals, but in captivity can do it for ten months on end, the whole of its life's span, apparently without inconvenience or fatigue.[1]

The fact is that when the mind is at rest nothing can tire the eyes, and when the mind is under a strain nothing can rest them. Anything that rests the mind will benefit the eyes. Almost everyone has observed that the eyes tire less quickly when reading an interesting book than when perusing something tiresome or difficult to comprehend. A schoolboy can sit up all night reading a novel without even thinking of his eyes, but if he tried to sit up all night studying his lessons he would soon find them getting very tired. A child whose vision was

---

[1] The Wonders of Instinct, English translation by de Mattos and Miall, 1918, pp. 36-38.

ordinarily so acute that she could see the moons of Jupiter with the naked eye became myopic when asked to do a sum in mental arithmetic, mathematics being a subject which was extremely distasteful to her. Sometimes the conditions which produce mental relaxation are very curious. One patient, for instance, was able to correct her error of refraction when she looked at the test card with her body bent over at an angle of about forty-five degrees, and the relaxation continued after she had assumed the upright position. Although the position was an unfavorable one, she had somehow got the idea that it improved her sight, and therefore it did so.

The time required to effect a permanent cure varies greatly with different individuals. In some cases five, ten, or fifteen minutes is sufficient, and I believe the time is coming when it will be possible to cure everyone quickly. It is only a question of accumulating more facts, and presenting these facts in such a way that the patient can grasp them quickly. At present, however, it is often necessary to continue the treatment for weeks and months, although the error of refraction may be no greater nor of longer duration than in those cases that are cured quickly. In most cases, too, the treatment must be continued for a few minutes every day to prevent relapse. Because a familiar object tends to relax the strain to see, the daily reading of the Snellen test card is usually sufficient for this purpose. It is also useful, particularly when the vision at the near point is imperfect, to read fine print every day as close to the eyes as it can be done. When a cure is complete it is always permanent; but complete cures, which mean the attainment, not of what is ordinarily called normal sight, but of a measure of telescopic and microscopic vision,

are very rare.   Even in these cases, too, the treatment
can be continued with benefit; for it is impossible to
place limits to the visual powers of man, and no matter
how good the sight, it is always possible to improve it.

Daily practice of the art of vision is also necessary to

Fig. 41.—One of Many Thousands of Patients Cured of Errors
of Refraction by the Methods Presented in This Book

No. 1.—Man of thirty-six, 1902, wearing glasses for myopia.
Note the appearance of effort in his eyes. He was relieved in
1904 by means of exercises in distant vision and obtained normal
sight without glasses.

No. 2.—The same man five years later. No relapse.

prevent those visual lapses to which every eye is liable,
no matter how good its sight may ordinarily be.   It is
true that no system of training will provide an absolute
safeguard against such lapses in all circumstances; but
the daily reading of small distant, familiar letters will
do much to lessen the tendency to strain when disturbing circumstances arise, and all persons upon whose eyesight the safety of others depends should be required
to do this.

Generally persons who have never worn glasses are

more easily cured than those who have, and glasses should be discarded at the beginning of the treatment. When this cannot be done without too great discomfort, or when the patient has to continue his work during the treatment and cannot do so without glasses, their use must be permitted for a time; but this always delays the cure. Persons of all ages have been benefited by this treatment of errors of refraction by relaxation; but children usually, though not invariably, respond much more quickly than adults. If they are under twelve years of age, or even under sixteen, and have never worn glasses, they are usually cured in a few days, weeks, or months, and always within a year, simply by reading the Snellen test card every day.

CHAPTER X

STRAIN

TEMPORARY conditions may contribute to the strain to see which results in the production of errors of refraction; but its foundation lies in wrong habits of thought. In attempting to relieve it the physician has continually to struggle against the idea that to do anything well requires effort. This idea is drilled into us from our cradles. The whole educational system is based upon it; and in spite of the wonderful results attained by Montessori through the total elimination of every species of compulsion in the educational process, educators who call themselves modern still cling to the club, under various disguises, as a necessary auxiliary to the process of imparting knowledge.

It is as natural for the eye to see as it is for the mind to acquire knowledge, and any effort in either case is not only useless, but defeats the end in view. You may force a few facts into a child's mind by various kinds of compulsion, but you cannot make it learn anything. The facts remain, if they remain at all, as dead lumber in the brain. They contribute nothing to the vital processes of thought; and because they were not acquired naturally and not assimilated, they destroy the natural impulse of the mind toward the acquisition of knowledge, and by the time the child leaves school or college, as the case may be, it not only knows nothing but is, in the majority of cases, no longer capable of learning.

In the same way you may temporarily improve the sight by effort, but you cannot improve it to normal, and if the effort is allowed to become continuous, the sight will steadily deteriorate and may eventually be destroyed. Very seldom is the impairment or destruction of vision due to any fault in the construction of the eye. Of two equally good pairs of eyes one will retain perfect sight to the end of life, and the other will lose it in the kindergarten, simply because one looks at things without effort and the other does not.

The eye with normal sight never tries to see. If for any reason, such as the dimness of the light, or the distance of the object, it cannot see a particular point, it shifts to another. It never tries to bring out the point by staring at it, as the eye with imperfect sight is constantly doing.

Whenever the eye tries to see, it at once ceases to have normal vision. A person may look at the stars with normal vision; but if he tries to count the stars in any particular constellation, he will probably become myopic. because the attempt to do these things usually results in an effort to see. A patient was able to look at the letter K on the Snellen test card with normal vision, but when asked to count its twenty-seven corners he lost it completely.

It obviously requires a strain to fail to see at the distance, because the eye at rest is adjusted for distant vision. If one does anything when one wants to see at the distance, one must do the wrong thing. The shape of the eyeball cannot be altered during distant vision without strain. It is equally a strain to fail to see at the near-point, because when the muscles respond to the mind's desire they do it without strain. Only by an effort can one prevent the eye from elongating at the near-point.

The eye possesses perfect vision only when it is absolutely at rest. Any movement, either in the organ or the object of vision, produces an error of refraction. With the retinoscope it can be demonstrated that even the necessary movements of the eyeball produce a slight error of refraction, and the moving pictures have given us a practical demonstration of the fact that it is impossible to see a moving object perfectly. When the movement of the object of vision is sufficiently slow, the resulting impairment of vision is so slight as to be inappreciable, just as the errors of refraction produced by slight movements of the eyeball are inappreciable; but when objects move very rapidly they can be seen only as a blur. For this reason it has been found necessary to arrange the machinery for exhibiting moving pictures in such a way that each picture is halted for a twenty-fourth of a second, and screened while it is moving into place. Moving pictures, accordingly, are never seen in motion.

The act of seeing is passive. Things are seen, just as they are felt, or heard, or tasted, without effort or volition on the part of the subject. When sight is perfect the letters on the test card are waiting, perfectly black and perfectly distinct, to be recognized. They do not have to be sought; they are there. In imperfect sight they are sought and chased. The eye goes after them. An effort is made to see them.

The muscles of the body are supposed never to be at rest. The blood-vessels, with their muscular coats, are never at rest. Even in sleep thought does not cease. But the normal condition of the nerves of sense—of hearing, sight, taste, smell and touch—is one of rest. They can be acted upon; they cannot act. The optic nerve, the retina and the visual centers of the brain are as passive as the finger-nail. They have nothing whatever in their structure that makes it possible for them to do anything, and when they are the subject of effort from outside sources their efficiency is always impaired.

The mind is the source of all such efforts from outside sources brought to bear upon the eye. Every thought of effort in the mind, of whatever sort, transmits a motor impulse to the eye; and every such impulse causes a deviation from the normal in the shape of the eyeball and lessens the sensitiveness of the center of sight. If one wants to have perfect sight, therefore, one must have no thought of effort in the mind. Mental strain of any kind always produces a conscious or unconscious eyestrain and if the strain takes the form of an effort to see, an error of refraction is always produced. A schoolboy was able to read the bottom line of the Snellen test card at ten feet, but when the teacher told him to mind what he was about he could not see the big C.[1] Many children can see perfectly so long as their mothers are around; but if the mother goes out of the room, they may at once become myopic, because of the strain produced by fear. Unfamiliar objects produce eyestrain and a consequent error of refraction, because they first produce mental strain. A person may have good vision when he is telling the truth; but if he states what is not true, even with no intent to deceive, or if he imagines what is not true, an error of refraction will be produced, because it is impossible to state or imagine what is not true without an effort.

I may claim to have discovered that telling lies is bad

---

[1] In this case and others to be mentioned later, the large letter at the top of the card read by the eye with normal vision at two hundred feet, was a "C."

for the eyes, and whatever bearing this circumstance may have upon the universality of defects of vision, the fact can easily be demonstrated. If a patient can read all the small letters on the bottom line of the test card, and either deliberately or carelessly miscalls any of them, the retinoscope will indicate an error of refraction. In numerous cases patients have been asked to state their ages incorrectly, or to try to imagine that they were a year older or a year younger than they actually were, and in every case when they did this the retinoscope indicated an error of refraction. A patient twenty-five years old had no error of refraction when he looked at a blank wall without trying to see; but if he said he was twenty-six or if someone else said he was twenty-six, or if he tried to imagine that he was twenty-six, he became myopic. The same thing happened when he stated or tried to imagine that he was twenty-four. When he stated or remembered the truth his vision was normal, but when he stated or imagined an error he had an error of refraction.

Two little girl patients arrived one after the other one day, and the first accused the second of having stopped at Huyler's for an ice cream soda, which she had been instructed not to do, being somewhat too much addicted to sweets. The second denied the charge, and the first, who had used the retinoscope and knew what it did to people who told lies, said:

"Do take the retinoscope and find out."

I followed the suggestion, and having thrown the light into the second child's eyes, I asked:

"Did you go to Huyler's?"

"Yes," was the response, and the retinoscope indicated no error of refraction.

"Did you have an ice-cream soda?"

"No," said the child; but the telltale shadow moved in a direction opposite to that of the mirror, showing that she had become myopic and was not telling the truth.

The child blushed when I told her this and acknowledged that the retinoscope was right; for she had heard of the ways of the uncanny instrument before and did not know what else it might do to her if she said anything more that was not true.

So sensitive is this test that if the subject. whether his vision is ordinarily normal or not, pronounces the initials of his name correctly while looking at a blank surface without trying to see, there will be no error of refraction; but if he miscalls one initial, even without any consciousness of effort, and with full knowledge that he is deceiving no one, myopia will be produced.

Mental strain may produce many different kinds of eyestrain. According to the statement of most authorities there is only one kind of eyestrain, an indefinite thing resulting from so-called over-use of the eyes, or an effort to overcome a wrong shape of the eyeball. It can be demonstrated, however, that there is not only a different strain for each different error of refraction, but a different strain for most abnormal conditions of the eye. The strain that produces an error of refraction is not the same as the strain that produces a squint, or a cataract,[1] or glaucoma,[2] or amblyopia,[3] or inflammation of the conjunctiva[4] or of the margin of the lids, or disease of the optic nerve or retina. All these conditions may exist

---

[1] An opacity of the lens.

[2] A condition in which the eyeball becomes abnormally hard.

[3] A condition in which there is a decline of vision without apparent cause.

[4] A membrane covering the inner surface of the eyelid and the visible part of the white of the eye.

with only a slight error of refraction, and while the relief
of one strain usually means the relief of any others that
may coexist with it, it sometimes happens that the strain
associated with such conditions as cataract and glaucoma is relieved without the complete relief of the strain
that causes the error of refraction. Even the pain that
so often accompanies errors of refraction is never caused
by the same strain that causes these errors. Some myopes cannot read without pain or discomfort, but most
of them suffer no inconvenience. When the hyperme-
trope regards an object at the distance the hypermetropia is lessened, but pain and discomfort may be increased. While there are many strains, however, there
is only one cure for all of them, namely, relaxation.

The health of the eye depends upon the blood, and
circulation is very largely influenced by thought. When
thought is normal—that is, not attended by any excitement or strain—the circulation in the brain is normal,
the supply of blood to the optic nerve and the visual
centers is normal. and the vision is perfect. When
thought is abnormal the circulation is disturbed, the
supply of blood to the optic nerve and visual centers is
altered, and the vision lowered. We can consciously
think thoughts which disturb the circulation and lower
the visual power; we can also consciously think thoughts
that will restore normal circulation, and thereby cure,
not only all errors of refraction, but many other abnormal conditions of the eyes. We cannot by any amount
of effort make ourselves see, but by learning to control
our thoughts we can accomplish that end indirectly.

You can teach people how to produce any error of
refraction, how to produce a squint, how to see two
images of an object, one above another, or side by side,

or at any desired angle from one another, simply by teaching them how to think in a particular way. When the disturbing thought is replaced by one that relaxes, the squint disappears, the double vision and the errors of refraction are corrected; and this is as true of abnormalties of long standing as of those produced voluntarily. No matter what their degree or their duration their cure is accomplished just as soon as the patient is able to secure mental control. The cause of any error of refraction, of a squint, or of any other functional disturbance of the eye, is simply a thought—a wrong thought—and the cure is as quick as the thought that relaxes. In a fraction of a second the highest degrees of refractive error may be corrected, a squint may disappear, or the blindness of amblyopia may be relieved. If the relaxation is only momentary, the correction is momentary. When it becomes permanent, the correction is permanent.

This relaxation cannot, however, be obtained by any sort of effort. It is fundamental that patients should understand this; for so long as they think, consciously or unconsciously, that relief from strain may be obtained by another strain their cure will be delayed.

CHAPTER XI

CENTRAL FIXATION

THE eye is a miniature camera, corresponding in many ways very exactly to the inanimate machine used in photography. In one respect, however, there is a great difference between the two instruments. The sensitive plate of the camera is equally sensitive in every part; but the retina has a point of maximum sensitiveness, and every other part is less sensitive in proportion as it is removed from that point. This point of maximum sensitiveness is called the "fovea centralis," literally the "central pit."

The retina, although it is an extremely delicate membrane, varying in thickness from one-eightieth of an inch to less than half that amount, is highly complex. It is composed of nine layers, only one of which is supposed to be capable of receiving visual impressions. This layer is composed of minute rodlike and conical bodies which vary in form and are distributed very differently in its different parts. In the center of the retina is a small circular elevation known, from the yellow color which it assumes in death and sometimes also in life, as the "macula lutea," literally the "yellow spot." In the center of this spot is the fovea, a deep depression of darker color. In the center of this depression there are no rods, and the cones are elongated and pressed very closely together. The other layers, on the contrary, become here extremely thin, or disappear altogether, so that the cones are covered with barely perceptible traces of them. Beyond the center of the fovea the cones become thicker and fewer and are interspersed with rods, the number of which increases toward the margin of the retina. The precise function of these rods and cones is not clear; but it is a fact that the center of the fovea, where all elements except the cones and their associated cells practically disappear, is the seat of the most acute vision. As we withdraw from this spot, the acuteness of the visual perceptions rapidly decreases. The eye with normal vision, therefore, sees one part of everything it looks at best, and everything else worse, in proportion as it is removed from the point of maximum vision; and it is an invariable symptom of all abnormal conditions of the eyes, both functional and organic, that this central fixation is lost.

These conditions are due to the fact that when the sight is normal the sensitiveness of the fovea is normal, but when the sight is imperfect, from whatever cause, the sensitiveness of the fovea is lowered, so that the eye sees equally well, or even better, with other parts of the retina. Contrary to what is generally believed, the part seen best when the sight is normal is extremely small. . The text-books say that at twenty feet an area having a diameter of half an inch can be seen with maximum vision, but anyone who tries at this distance to see every part of even the smallest letters of the Snellen test card—the diameter of which may be less than a quarter of an inch—equally well at one time will immediately become myopic. The fact is that the nearer the point of maximum vision approaches a mathematical point, which has no area, the better the sight.

The cause of this loss of function in the center of sight is mental strain; and as all abnormal conditions of the eyes, organic as well as functional, are accompanied by mental strain, all such conditions must necessarily be accompanied by loss of central fixation. When the mind is under a strain the eye usually goes more or less blind. The center of sight goes blind first, partially or completely, according to the degree of the strain, and if the strain is great enough the whole or the greater part of the retina may be involved. When the vision of the center of sight has been suppressed, partially or completely, the patient can no longer see the point which he is looking at best, but sees objects not regarded directly as well, or better, because the sensitiveness of the retina has now become approximately equal in every part, or is even better in the outer part than in the center. Therefore in all cases of defective vision the patient is unable to see best where he is looking.

This condition is sometimes so extreme that the patient may look as far away from an object as it is possible to see it, and yet see it just as well as when looking directly at it. In one case it had gone so far that the patient could see only with the edge of the retina on the nasal side. In other words, she could not see her fingers in front of her face, but could see them if held at the outer side of her eye. She had only a slight error of refraction, showing that while every error of refraction is accompanied by eccentric fixation, the strain which causes the one condition is different from that which produces the other. The patient had been examined by specialists in this country and Europe, who attributed her blindness to disease of the optic nerve or brain; but the fact that vision was restored by relaxation demonstrated that the condition had been due simply to mental strain.

Eccentric fixation, even in its lesser degrees, is so unnatural that great discomfort, or even pain, can be produced in a few seconds by trying to see every part of an area three or four inches in extent at twenty feet, or even less, or an area of an inch or less at the near-point, equally well at one time, while at the same time the retinoscope will demonstrate that an error of refraction has been produced. This strain, when it is habitual, leads to all sorts of abnormal conditions and is, in fact, at the bottom of most eye troubles, both functional and organic. The discomfort and pain may be absent, however, in the chronic condition, and it is an encouraging symptom when the patient begins to experience them.

When the eye possesses central fixation it not only possesses perfect sight, but it is perfectly at rest and can be used indefinitely without fatigue. It is open and quiet; no nervous movements are observable; and when it regards a point at the distance the visual axes are parallel. In other words, there are no muscular insufficiencies. This fact is not generally known. The textbooks state that muscular insufficiencies occur in eyes having normal sight, but I have never seen such a case. The muscles of the face and of the whole body are also at rest, and when the condition is habitual there are no wrinkles or dark circles around the eyes.

In most cases of eccentric fixation, on the contrary, the eye quickly tires, and its appearance, with that of the face, is expressive of effort or strain. The ophthalmoscope[1] reveals that the eyeball moves at irregular intervals, from side to side, vertically or in other directions. These movements are often so extensive as to be manifest by ordinary inspection, and are sometimes sufficiently marked to resemble nystagmus.[2] Nervous move-

---

[1] A shorter movement can be noted when the observer watches the optic nerve with the ophthalmoscope than when he views merely the exterior of the eye.

[2] A condition in which there is a conspicuous and more or less rhythmic movement of the eyeball from side to side.

ments of the eyelids may also be noted, either by ordinary inspection, or by lightly touching the lid of one eye while the other regards an object either at the near-point or the distance. The visual axes are never parallel, and the deviation from the normal may become so marked as to constitute the condition of squint. Redness of the conjunctiva and of the margins of the lids, wrinkles around the eyes, dark circles beneath them and tearing are other symptoms of eccentric fixation.

Eccentric fixation is a symptom of strain, and is relieved by any method that relieves strain; but in some cases the patient is cured just as soon as he is able to demonstrate the facts of central fixation. When he comes to realize, through actual demonstration of the fact, that he does not see best where he is looking, and that when he looks a sufficient distance away from a point he can see it worse than when he looks directly at it, he becomes able, in some way, to reduce the distance to which he has to look in order to see worse, until he can look directly at the top of a small letter and see the bottom worse, or look at the bottom and see the top worse. The smaller the letter regarded in this way, or the shorter the distance the patient has to look away from a letter in order to see the opposite part indistinctly, the greater the relaxation and the better the sight. When it becomes possible to look at the bottom of a letter and see the top worse, or to look at the top and see the bottom worse, it becomes possible to see the letter perfectly black and distinct. At first such vision may come only in flashes. The letter will come out distinctly for a moment and then disappear. But gradually, if the practice is continued, central fixation will become habitual.

Most patients can readily look at the bottom of the

big C and see the top worse; but in some cases it is not only impossible for them to do this, but impossible for them to let go of the large letters at any distance at which they can be seen. In these extreme cases it sometimes requires considerable ingenuity, first to demonstrate to the patient that he does not see best where he is looking, and then to help him to see an object worse when he looks away from it than when he looks directly at it. The use of a strong light as one of the points of fixation, or of two lights five or ten feet apart, has been found helpful, the patient when he looks away from the light being able to see it less bright more readily than he can see a black letter worse when he looks away from it. It then becomes easier for him to see the letter worse when he looks away from it. This method was successful in the following case:

A patient with vision of 3/200, when she looked at a point a few feet away from the big C, said she saw the letter better than when she looked directly at it. Her attention was called to the fact that her eyes soon became tired and that her vision soon failed when she saw things in this way. Then she was directed to look at a bright object about three feet away from the card, and this attracted her attention to such an extent that she became able to see the large letter on the test card worse, after which she was able to look back at it and see it better. It was demonstrated to her that she could do one of two things: look away and see the letter better than she did before, or look away and see it worse. She then became able to see it worse all the time when she looked three feet away from it. Next she became able to shorten the distance successively to two feet, one foot, and six inches, with a constant improvement in vision; and finally she became able to look at the bottom of the letter and see the top worse, or look at the top and see the bottom worse. With practice she became able to look at the smaller letters in the same way, and finally she became able to read the ten line at twenty feet. By the same method also she became able to read diamond type, first at twelve inches and then at three inches. By these simple measures alone she became able, in short, to see best where she was looking, and her cure was complete.

The highest degrees of eccentric fixation occur in the high degrees of myopia, and in these cases, since the sight is best at the near-point, the patient is benefited by practicing seeing worse at this point. The distance can then be gradually extended until it becomes possible to do the same thing at twenty feet. One patient with a high degree of myopia said that the farther she looked away from an electric light the better she saw it, but by alternately looking at the light at the near-point and looking away from it she became able, in a short time, to see it brighter when she looked directly at it than when she looked away from it. Later she became able to do the same thing at twenty feet, and then she experienced a wonderful feeling of relief. No words, she said, could adequately describe it. Every nerve seemed to be relaxed, and a feeling of comfort and rest permeated her whole body. Afterward her progress was rapid. She soon became able to look at one part of the smallest letters on the card and see the rest worse, and then she became able to read the letters at twenty feet.

On the principle that a burnt child dreads the fire, some patients are benefited by consciously making their sight worse. When they learn, by actual demonstration of the facts, just how their visual defects are produced, they **unconsciously** avoid the unconscious strain which causes them. When the degree of eccentric fixation is not too extreme to be increased, therefore, it is a benefit to patients to teach them how to increase it. When a patient has consciously lowered his vision and produced discomfort and even pain by trying to see the big C, or a whole line of letters, equally well at one time, he becomes better able to correct the unconscious effort of the eye to see all parts of a smaller area equally well at one time.

In learning to see best where he is looking it is usually best for the patient to think of the point not directly regarded as being seen less distinctly than the point he is looking at, instead of thinking of the point fixed as being seen best, as the latter practice has a tendency, in most cases, to intensify the strain under which the eye is already laboring. One part of an object is seen best only when the mind is content to see the greater part of it indistinctly, and as the degree of relaxation increases the area of the part seen worse increases, until that seen best becomes merely a point.

The limits of vision depend upon the degree of central fixation. A person may be able to read a sign half a mile away when he sees the letters all alike, but when taught to see one letter best he will be able to read smaller letters that he didn't know were there. The remarkable vision of savages, who can see with the naked eye objects for which most civilized persons require a telescope, is a matter of central fixation. Some people can see the rings of Saturn, or the moons of Jupiter, with the naked eye. It is not because of any superiority in the structure of their eyes, but because they have attained a higher degree of central fixation than most civilized persons do.

Not only do all errors of refraction and all functional

disturbances of the eye disappear when it sees by central fixation, but many organic conditions are relieved or cured. I am unable to set any limits to its possibilities. I would not have ventured to predict that glaucoma, incipient cataract and syphilitic iritis could be cured by central fixation; but it is a fact that these conditions have disappeared when central fixation was attained. Relief was often obtained in a few minutes, and, in rare cases, this relief was permanent. Usually, however, a permanent cure required more prolonged treatment. Inflammatory conditions of all kinds, including inflammation of the cornea, iris, conjunctiva, the various coats of the eyeball and even the optic nerve itself, have been benefited by central fixation after other methods had failed. Infections, as well as diseases caused by protein poisoning and the poisons of typhoid fever, influenza, syphilis and gonorrhœa, have also been benefited by it. Even with a foreign body in the eye there is no redness and no pain so long as central fixation is retained.

Since central fixation is impossible without mental control, central fixaton of the eye means central fixation of the mind. It means, therefore, health in all parts of the body, for all the operations of the physical mechanism depend upon the mind. Not only the sight, but all the other senses—touch, taste, hearing and smell—are benefited by central fixation. All the vital processes—digesttion, assimilation, elimination, etc.—are improved by it. The symptoms of functional and organic diseases are relieved. The efficiency of the mind is enormously increased. The benefits of central fixation already observed are, in short, so great that the subject merits further investigation.

CHAPTER XII

PALMING

ALL the methods used in the cure of errors of refraction are simply different ways of obtaining relaxation, and most patients, though by no means all, find it easiest to relax with their eyes shut. This usually lessens the strain to see, and in such cases is followed by a temporary or more lasting improvement in vision.

Most patients are benefited merely by closing the eyes; and by alternately resting them for a few minutes or longer in this way and then opening them and looking at the Snellen test card for a second or less, flashes of improved vision are, as a rule, very quickly obtained. Some temporarily obtain almost normal vision by this means; and in rare cases a complete cure has been effected, sometimes in less than an hour.

But since some light comes through the closed eyelids, a still greater degree of relaxation can be obtained, in all but a few exceptional cases, by excluding it. This is done by covering the closed eyes with the palms of the hands (the fingers being crossed upon the forehead) in such a way as to avoid pressure on the eyeballs. So efficacious is this practice, which I have called "palming," as a means of relieving strain, that we all instinctively resort to it at times, and from it most patients are able to get a considerable degree of relaxation.

But even with the eyes closed and covered in such a way as to exclude all the light, the visual centers of the brain may still be disturbed, the eye may still strain to see; and instead of seeing a field so black that it is impossible to remember, imagine, or see anything blacker, as one ought normally to do when the optic nerve is not subject to the stimulation of light, the patient will see illusions of lights and colors ranging all the way from an imperfect black to kaleidoscopic appearances so vivid that they seem to be actually seen with the eyes. The worse the condition of the eyesight, as a rule, the more numerous, vivid and persistent these appearances are. Yet some persons with very imperfect sight are able to palm almost perfectly from the beginning, and are, therefore, very quickly cured. Any disturbance of mind or body, such as fatigue, hunger, anger, worry or depression, also makes it difficult for patients to see black when they palm, persons who can see it perfectly under ordinary conditions being often unable to do so without assistance when they are ill or in pain.

It is impossible to see a perfect black unless the eyesight is perfect, because only when the eyesight is perfect is the mind at rest; but some patients can without difficulty approximate such a black nearly enough to improve their eyesight, and as the eyesight improves the deepness of the black increases. Patients who fail to see even an approximate black when they palm state that instead of black they see streaks or floating clouds of gray, flashes of light, patches of red, blue, green, yellow, etc. Sometimes instead of an immovable black, clouds of black will be seen moving across the field. In other cases the black will be seen for a few seconds and then some other color will take its place. The different ways in which patients can fail to see black when their eyes are closed and covered are, in fact, very numerous and often very peculiar.

Some patients have been so impressed with the vividness of the colors which they imagined they saw that no amount of argument could, or did, convince them that they did not actually see them with their eyes. If

Fig. 42. Palming

This is one of the most effective methods of obtaining relaxation of all the sensory nerves.

other people saw bright lights or colors, with their eyes closed and covered, they admitted that these things would be illusions; but what they themselves saw under the same conditions was reality. They would not believe, until they had themselves demonstrated the truth, that their illusions were due to an imagination beyond their control.

Successful palming in these more difficult cases usually involves the practice of all the methods for improving the sight described in succeeding chapters. For reasons which will be explained in the following chapter, the majority of such patients may be greatly helped by the memory of a black object. They are directed to look at such an object at the distance at which the color can be seen best, close the eyes and remember the color, and repeat until the memory appears to be equal to the sight. Then they are instructed, while still holding the memory of the black, to cover the closed eyes with the palms of the hands in the manner just described. If the memory of the black is perfect, the whole background will be black. If it is not, or if it does not become so in the course of a few seconds, the eyes are opened and the black object regarded again.

Many patients become able by this method to see black almost perfectly for a short time; but most of them, even those whose eyes are not very bad, have great difficulty in seeing it continuously. Being unable to remember black for more than from three to five seconds, they cannot see black for a longer time than this. Such patients are helped by central fixation. When they have become able to see one part of a black object darker than the whole, they are able to remember the smaller area for a longer time than they could the larger one, and thus become able to see black for a longer period when they palm. They are also benefited by mental shifting (see Chapter XV) from one black object to another, or from one part of a black object to another. It is impossible to see, remember, or imagine anything, even for as much as a second, without shifting from one part to another, or to some other object and back again; and the attempt to do so always produces strain. Those who think they are remembering a black object continuously are unconsciously comparing it with something not so black, or

Fig. 43

Patient with atrophy of the optic nerve gets flashes of improved vision after palming.

else its color and its position are constantly changing. It is impossible to remember even such a simple thing as a period perfectly black and stationary for more than a fraction of a second. When shifting is not done unconsciously patients must be encouraged to do it consciously. They may be directed, for instance, to remember successively a black hat, a black shoe, a black velvet dress, a black plush curtain, or a fold in the black dress or the black curtain, holding each one not more than a fraction of a second. Many persons have been benefited by remembering all the letters of the alphabet in turn perfectly black. Others prefer to shift from one small black object, such as a period or a small letter, to another, or to swing such an object in a manner to be described later (see Chapter XV).

In some cases the following method has proved successful: When the patient sees what he thinks is a perfect black, let him remember a piece of starch on this background, and on the starch the letter F as black as the background. Then let him let go of the starch and remember only the F, one part best, on the black background. In a short time the whole field may become as black as the blacker part of the F. The process can be repeated many times with a constant increase of blackness in the field.

In one case a patient who saw grey so vividly when she palmed that she was positive she saw it with her eyes, instead of merely imagining it, was able to obliterate nearly all of it by first imagining a black C on the grey field, then two black C's, and finally a multitude of overlapping C's.

It is impossible to remember black perfectly when it is not seen perfectly. If one sees it imperfectly, the best one can do is to remember it imperfectly. All persons, without exception, who can see or read diamond type at the near-point, no matter how great their myopia may be, or how much the interior of the eye may be diseased, become able, as a rule, to see black with their eyes closed and covered more readily than patients with hypermetropia or astigmatism; because, while myopes cannot see anything perfectly, even at the near-point, they see better at that point than persons with hypermetropia or astigmatism do at any distance. Persons with high degrees of myopia, however, often find palming very difficult, since they not only see black very imperfectly, but, because of the effort they are making to see, cannot remember it more than one or two seconds. Any other condition of the eye which prevents the patient from seeing black perfectly also makes palming difficult. In some cases black is never seen as black, appearing to be grey, yellow, brown, or even bright red. In such cases it is usually best for the patient to improve his sight by other methods before trying to palm. Blind persons usually have more trouble in seeing black than those who can see, but may be helped by the memory of a black object familiar to them before they lost their sight. A blind painter who saw grey continually when he first tried to palm became able at last to see black by the aid of the memory of black paint. He had no perception of light whatever and was in terrible pain; but when he succeeded in seeing black the pain vanished, and when he opened his eyes he saw light.

Even the imperfect memory of black is useful, for by its aid a still blacker black can be both remembered and seen; and this brings still further improvement. For instance, let the patient regard a letter on the Snellen test card at the distance at which the color is seen best, then close his eyes and remember it. If the palming produces relaxation, it will be possible to imagine a deeper shade of black than was seen, and by remembering this black when again regarding the letter it can be seen blacker than it was at first. A still deeper black can then be imagined, and this deeper black can, in turn, be transferred to the letter on the test card. By continuing this process a perfect perception of black, and hence perfect sight, are sometimes very quickly obtained. The deeper the shade of black obtained with the eyes closed, the more easily it can be remembered when regarding the letters on the test card.

The longer some people palm the greater the relaxation they obtain and the darker the shade of black they are able both to remember and see. Others are able to palm successfully for short periods, but begin to strain if they keep it up too long.

It is impossible to succeed by effort, or by attempting to "concentrate" on the black. As popularly understood, concentration means to do or think one thing only; but this is impossible, and an attempt to do the impossible is a strain which defeats its own end. The human mind is not capable of thinking of one thing only. It can think of one thing best, and is only at rest when it does so; but it cannot think of one thing only. A patient who tried to see black only and to ignore the kaleidoscopic colors which intruded themselves upon her field of vision, becoming worse and worse the more they were ignored, actually went into convulsions from the strain, and was attended every day for a month by her family physician before she was able to resume the treatment. This patient was advised to stop palming, and, with her eyes open, to recall as many colors as possible, remembering each one as perfectly as possible. By thus taking the bull by the horns and consciously making the mind wander more than it did unconsciously, she became able, in some way, to palm for short periods.

Some particular kinds of black objects may be found to be more easily remembered than others. Black plush of a high grade for instance, proved to be an optimum (see Chapter XVIII) with many persons as compared with black velvet, silk, broadcloth, ink and the letters on the Snellen test card, although no blacker than these other blacks. A familiar black object can often be remembered more easily by the patient than those that

Fig. 44

No. 1.—Owing to paralysis of the seventh nerve on the right side, resulting from a mastoid operation on the right ear, the patient is unable to close her lips.

No. 2.—After palming and remembering a perfectly black period she became able not only to close the lips, but to whistle. The cure was permanent.

are less so. A dressmaker, for instance, was able to remember a thread of black silk when she could not remember any other black object.

When a black letter is regarded before palming the patient will usually remember not only the blackness of the letter, but the white background as well. If the memory of the black is held for a few seconds, however, the background usually fades away and the whole field becomes black.

Patients often say that they remember black perfectly when they do not. One can usually tell whether or not this is the case by noting the effect of palming upon the vision. If there is no improvement in the sight when the eyes are opened, it can be demonstrated, by bringing the black closer to the patient, that it has not been remembered perfectly.

Although black is, as a rule, the easiest color to remember, for reasons explained in the next chapter, the following method sometimes succeeds when the memory of black fails: Remember a variety of colors—bright red, yellow, green, blue, purple, white especially—all in the most intense shade possible. Do not attempt to hold any of them more than a second. Keep this up for five or ten minutes. Then remember a piece of starch about half an inch in diameter as white as possible. Note the color of the background. Usually it will be a shade of black. If it is, note whether it is possible to remember anything blacker, or to see anything blacker with the eyes open. In all cases when the white starch is remembered perfectly the background will be so black that it will be impossible to remember anything blacker with the eyes closed, or to see anything blacker with them open.

When palming is successful it is one of the best methods I know of for securing relaxation of all the sensory nerves, including those of sight. When perfect relaxation is gained in this way, as indicated by the ability to see a perfect black, it is completely retained when the eyes are opened, and the patient is permanently cured. At the same time pain in the eyes and head, and even in other parts of the body, is permanently relieved. Such cases are very rare, but they do occur. With a lesser

Fig 45

Fig. 1.—Patient with absolute glaucoma of the right eye. He had suffered agonizing pain for six months and had no perception of light. He was photographed when testing the tension of his eyeball, which he found to be perfectly hard.

Fig. 2.—The patient is palming and remembering a perfectly black period. After half an hour the eyeball became soft, the pain ceased, and the patient became able to see the light. After three years there was no return of the glaucoma.

degree of relaxation much of it is lost when the eyes are opened, and what is retained is not held permanently. In other words, the greater the degree of the relaxation produced by palming the more of it is retained when the eyes are opened and the longer it lasts. If you palm perfectly, you retain, when you open your eyes, all of the relaxation that you gain, and you do not lose it again. If you palm imperfectly, you retain only part of what you gain and retain it only temporarily—it may be only for a few moments. Even the smallest degree of relaxation is useful, however, for by means of it a still greater degree may be obtained.

Patients who succeed with palming from the beginning are to be congratulated, for they are always cured very quickly. A very remarkable case of this kind was that of a man nearly seventy years of age with compound hypermetropic astigmatism and presbyopia, complicated by incipient cataract. For more than forty years he had worn glasses to improve his distant vision, and for twenty years he had worn them for reading and desk work. Because of the cloudiness of the lens, he had now become unable to see well enough to do his work, even with glasses; and the other physicians whom he had consulted had given him no hope of relief except by operation when the cataract was ripe. When he found palming helped him, he asked:

"Can I do that too much?"

"No," he was told. "Palming is simply a means of resting your eyes, and you cannot rest them too much."

A few days later he returned and said:

"Doctor, it was tedious, very tedious; but I did it."

"What was tedious?" I asked.

"Palming," he replied. "I did it continuously for twenty hours."

"But you couldn't have kept it up for twenty hours continuously," I said incredulously. "You must have stopped to eat."

And then he related that from four o'clock in the morning until twelve at night he had eaten nothing, only drinking large quantities of water, and had devoted practically all of the time to palming. It must have been tedious, as he said, but it was also worth while. When he looked at the test card, without glasses, he read the bottom line at twenty feet. He also read fine print at six inches and at twenty. The cloudiness of the lens had become much less, and in the center had entirely disappeared. Two years later there had been no relapse.

Although the majority of patients are helped by palming, a minority are unable to see black, and only increase their strain by trying to get relaxation in this way. In most cases it is possible, by using some or all of the various methods outlined in this chapter, to enable the patient to palm successfully; but if much difficulty is experienced, it is usually better and more expeditious to drop the method until the sight has been improved by other means. The patient may then become able to see black when he palms, but some never succeed in doing it until they are cured.

CHAPTER XIII

MEMORY AS AN AID TO VISION

WHEN the mind is able to remember perfectly any phenomenon of the senses, it is always perfectly relaxed. The sight is normal, if the eyes are open; and when they are closed and covered so as to exclude all the light, one sees a perfectly black field —that is nothing at all. If you can remember the ticking of a watch, or an odor or a taste perfectly, your mind is perfectly at rest, and you will see a perfect black when your eyes are closed and covered. If your memory of a sensation of touch could be equal to the reality, you would see nothing but black when the light was excluded from your eyes. If you were to remember a bar of music perfectly when your eyes were closed and covered, you would see nothing but black. But in the case of any of these phenomena it is not easy to test the correctness of the memory, and the same is true of colors other than black. All other colors, including white, are altered by the amount of light to which they are exposed, and are seldom seen as perfectly as it is possible for the normal eye to see them. But when the sight is normal, black is just as black in a dim light as in a bright one. It is also just as black at the distance as at the near-point, while a small area is just as black as a large one, and, in fact, appears blacker. Black is, moreover, more readily available than any other color. There is nothing blacker than printer's ink, and that is practically ubiquitous. By means of the memory of black, therefore, it is possible to measure accurately one's own relaxation. If the color is remembered perfectly, one is perfectly relaxed. If it is remembered almost perfectly, one's relaxation is almost perfect. If it cannot be remembered at all, one has very little or no relaxation.

By means of simultaneous retinoscopy, these facts can be readily demonstrated. An absolutely perfect memory is very rare, so much so that it need hardly be taken into consideration; but a practically perfect memory, or what might be called normal, is attainable by every one under certain conditions. With such a memory of black, the retinoscope shows that all errors of refraction are corrected. If the memory is less than normal, the contrary will be the case. If it fluctuates, the shadow of the retinoscope will fluctuate. The testimony of the retinoscope is, in fact, more reliable than the statements of the patient. Patients often believe and state that they remember black perfectly, or normally, when the retinoscope indicates an error of refraction; but in such cases it can usually be demonstrated by bringing the test card to the point at which the black letters can be seen best, that the memory is not equal to the sight. That the color cannot be remembered perfectly when the eyes and mind are under a strain, the reader can easily demonstrate by trying to remember it when making a conscious effort to see—by staring, partly closing the eyes, frowning, etc.—or while trying to see all the letters of a line equally well at one time. It will be found that it either cannot be remembered at all under these conditions, or that it is remembered very imperfectly.

When the two eyes of a patient are different, it has been found that the difference can be exactly measured by the length of time a black period can be remembered, while looking at the Snellen test card, with both eyes open, and with the better eye closed. A patient with normal vision in the right eye and half-normal vision in the left could, when looking at the test card with both eyes open, remember a period for twenty seconds continuously; but with the better eye closed, it could be remembered only ten seconds. A patient with half-normal vision in the right eye and one-quarter normal in the left could remember a period twelve seconds with both eyes open, and only six seconds with the better eye closed. A third patient, with normal sight in the right eye and vision of one-tenth in the left, could remember a period twenty seconds with both eyes open, and only two seconds when the better eye was closed. In other words, if the right eye is better than the left, the memory is better when the right eye is open than when only the left eye is open, the difference being in exact proportion to the difference in the vision of the two eyes.

In the treatment of functional eye troubles this relationship between relaxation and memory is of great practical importance. The sensations of the eye and of the mind supply very little information as to the strain to which both are being subjected, those who strain most often suffering the least discomfort; but by means of his ability to remember black the patient can always know whether he is straining or not, and is able, therefore, to avoid the conditions that produce strain. Whatever method of improving his sight the patient is using, he is advised to carry with him constantly the memory of a small area of black, such as a period, so that

he may recognize and avoid the conditions that produce strain, and in some cases patients have obtained a
complete cure in a very short time by this means alone.
One advantage of the method is that it does not require a
test card, for at any hour of the day or night, whatever the patient may be doing, he can always place himself in the conditions favorable to the perfect memory of
a period.

The condition of mind in which a black period can
be remembered cannot be attained by any sort of effort.
The memory is not the cause of the relaxation, but must
be preceded by it. It is obtained only during moments
of relaxation, and retained only as long as the causes
of strain are avoided; but how this is accomplished cannot be fully explained, just as many other psychological
phenomena cannot be explained. We only know that
under certain conditions that might be called favorable
a degree of relaxation sufficient for the memory of a
black period is possible, and that, by persistently seeking these conditions, the patient becomes able to increase
the degree of the relaxation and prolong its duration,
and finally becomes able to retain it under unfavorable
conditions.

For most patients palming provides the most favorable conditions for the memory of black. When the
strain to see is lessened by the exclusion of the light,
the patient usually becomes able to remember a black
object for a few seconds or longer, and this period of
relaxation can be prolonged in one of two ways. Either
the patient can open his eyes and look at a black object
by central fixation at the distance at which it can be
seen best, and at which the eyes are, therefore, most
relaxed, or he can shift mentally from one black object to

another, or from one part of a black object to another. By these means, and perhaps also through other influences that are not clearly understood, most patients become able, sooner or later, to remember black for an indefinite length of time with their eyes closed and covered.

With the eyes open and looking at a blank surface without trying consciously to see, the unconscious strain is lessened so that the patient becomes able to remember a black period, and all errors of refraction, as demonstrated by the retinoscope, are corrected. This result has been found to be invariable, and so long as the surface remains blank and the patient does not begin to remember or imagine things seen imperfectly, the memory and the vision may be retained. But if, with the improved vision, details upon the surface begin to come out, or if the patient begins to think of the test card, which he has seen imperfectly, the strain to see will return and the period will be lost.

When looking at a surface on which there is nothing particular to see, distance makes no difference to the memory, because the patient can always look at such a surface, no matter where it is, without straining to see it. When looking at letters, or other details, however, the memory is best at the point at which the patient's sight is best, because at that point the eyes and mind are more relaxed than when the same letters or objects are regarded at distances at which the vision is not so good. By practicing central fixation at the most favorable distance, therefore, and using any other means of improving the vision which are found effectual, the memory of the period may be improved, in some cases, very rapidly.

If the relaxation gained under these favorable conditions is perfect, the patient will be able to retain it when the mind is conscious of the impressions of sight at unfavorable distances. Such cases are, however, very rare. Usually the degree of relaxation gained is markedly imperfect, and is, therefore, lost to a greater or less degree when the conditions are unfavorable, as when letters or objects are being regarded at unfavorable distances. So disturbing are the impressions of sight under these circumstances, that just as soon as details begin to come out at distances at which they have not previously been seen, the patient usually loses his relaxation, and with it the memory of the period. In fact, the strain to see may even return before he has had time to become conscious of the image on his retina, as the following case strikingly illustrates:

A woman of fifty-five who had myopia of fifteen diopters, complicated with other conditions which made it impossible for her to see the big C at more than one foot, or to go about, either in her house or on the street, without an attendant, became able, when she looked at a green wall without trying to see it, to remember a perfectly black period and to see a small area of the wall-paper at the distance as well as she could at the near-point. When she had come close to the wall, she was asked to put her hand on the door-knob, which she did without hesitation. "But I don't see the knob," she hastened to explain. As a matter of fact she had seen it long enough to put her hand on it; but as soon as the idea of seeing it was suggested to her she lost the memory of the period, and with it her improved vision, and when she again tried to find the knob she could not do so.

When a period is remembered perfectly while a let-

ter on the Snellen test card is being regarded, the letter improves, with or without the consciousness of the
patient; because it is impossible to strain and relax at
the same time, and if one relaxes sufficiently to remember the period, one must also relax sufficiently to see the
letter, consciously or unconsciously.   Letters on either
side of the one regarded, or on the lines above and below
it, also improve.   When the patient is conscious of seeing the letters, this is very distracting, and usually
causes him, at first, to forget the period; while with some
patients, as already noted, the strain may return even
before the letters are consciously recognized.

Thus patients find themselves on the horns of a
dilemma.   The relaxation indicated by the memory of a
period improves their sight, and the things they see
with this improved vision cause them to lose their relaxation and their memory.   It is very remarkable to me
how the difficulty is ever overcome, but some patients
are able to do it in five minutes or half an hour.   With
others the process is long and tedious.

There are various ways of helping patients to deal with
this situation.   One is to direct them to remember the
period while looking a little to one side of the test card,
say a foot or more; then to look a little nearer to it, and
finally to look between the lines.   In this way they may
become able to see the letters in the eccentric field without losing the period; and when they can do this they
may become able to go a step farther, and look directly
at a letter without losing control of their memory.   If
they cannot do it, they are told to look at only one part
of a letter—usually the bottom—or to see or imagine the
period as part of the letter, while noting that the rest
of the letter is less black and less distinct than the part

directly regarded. When they can do this they become able to remember the period better than when the letter is seen all alike. If the letter is seen all alike, the perfect memory of the period is always lost. The next step is to ask the patient to note whether the bottom of the letter is straight, curved, or open, without losing the period on the bottom. When he can do this, he is asked to do the same with the sides and top of the letter, still holding the period on the bottom. Usually when the parts can be observed separately in this way, the whole letter can be seen without losing the memory of the period; but it occasionally happens that this is not the case, and further practice is needed before the patient can become conscious of all sides of the letter at once without losing the period. This may require moments, hours, days, or months. In one case the following method succeeded:

The patient, a man with fifteen diopters of myopia, was so much disturbed by what he saw when his vision had been improved by the memory of a period that he was directed to look away from the Snellen test card, or whatever object he was regarding, when he found the letters or other details coming out; and for about a week he went around persistently dodging his improved sight. As his memory improved, it became more and more difficult for him to do this, and at the end of the week it was impossible. When he looked at the bottom line at a distance of twenty feet he remembered the period perfectly, and when asked if he could see the letters, he replied:

"I cannot help but see them."

Some patients retard their recovery by decorating the scenery with periods as they go about during the day, instead of simply remembering a period in their minds. This does them no good, but is, on the contrary, a cause of strain. The period can be imagined perfectly and with benefit as forming part of a black letter on the test card, because this merely means imagining that one sees one part of the black letter best; but it cannot be imagined perfectly on any surface which is not black, and to attempt to imagine it on such surfaces defeats the end in view.

The smaller the area of black which the patient is able to remember, the greater is the degree of relaxation indicated; but some patients find it easier, at first, to remember a somewhat larger area, such as one of the letters on the Snellen test card with one part blacker than the rest. They may begin with the big C, then proceed to the smaller letters, and finally get to a period. It is then found that this small area is remembered more easily than the larger ones, and that its black is more intense. Instead of a period, some patients find it easier to remember a colon, with one period blacker than the other, or a collection of periods, with one blacker than all the others, or the dot over an i or j. Others, again, prefer a comma to a period. In the beginning most patients find it helpful to shift consciously from one of these black areas to another, or from one part of such an area to another, and to realize the swing, or pulsation, produced by such shifting (see Chapter XV); but when the memory becomes perfect, one object may be held continuously, without conscious shifting, while the swing is realized only when attention is directed to the matter.

Although black is, as a rule, the best color to remember, some patients are bored or depressed by it, and prefer to remember white or some other color. A familiar object, or one with pleasant associations, is often easier to remember than one which has no particular interest. One patient was cured by the memory of a yellow buttercup, and another was able to remember the opal of her ring when she could not remember a period. Whatever the patient finds easiest to remember is the best to remember, because the memory can never be perfect unless it is easy.

When the memory of the period becomes habitual, it is not only not a burden, but is a great help to other mental processes. Then mind, when it remembers one thing better than all other things, possesses central fixation, and its efficiency is thereby increased, just as the efficiency of the eye is increased by central fixation. In other words, the mind attains its greatest efficiency when it is at rest, and it is never at rest unless one thing is remembered better than all other things. When the mind is in such a condition that a period is remembered perfectly, the memory for other things is improved.

A high-school girl reports that when she was unable to remember the answer to a question in an examination, she remembered the period, and the answer came to her. When I cannot remember the name of a patient, I remember a period—and, behold, I have it! A musician who had perfect sight and could remember a period perfectly, had a perfect memory for music; but a musician with imperfect sight who could not remember a period could play nothing without his notes, only gaining that power when his sight and visual memory had become normal. In some exceptional cases, the strain to see letters on the Snellen test card has been so terrific that patients have said that they not only could not remember a period while they were looking at them, but could not remember even their own names.

Patients may measure the accuracy of their memory of the period, not only by comparing it with the sight, but by the following tests:

When the memory of the period is perfect it is instantaneous. If a few seconds or longer are necessary to obtain the memory, it is never perfect.

A perfect memory is not only instantaneous, but continuous.

When the period is remembered perfectly perfect sight comes instantaneously. If good vision is obtained only after a second or two, it can always be demonstrated that the memory of the period is imperfect and the sight also.

The memory of a period is a test of relaxation. It is the evidence by which the patient knows that his eyes and mind are at rest. It may be compared to the steam-gauge of an engine, which has nothing to do with the machinery, but is of great importance in giving information as to the ability of the mechanism to do its work. When the period is black one knows that the engine of the eye is in good working order. When the period fades, or is lost, one knows that it is out of order, until a cure is effected. Then one does not need a period, or any other aid to vision, just as the engineer does not need a steam-gauge when the engine is going properly. One patient who had gained telescopic and microscopic vision by the methods presented in this book said, in answer to an inquiry from some one interested in investigating the treatment of errors of refraction without glasses, that he had not only done nothing to prevent a relapse. but had even forgotten how he was cured.

The reply was unsatisfactory to the inquirer, but is quoted to illustrate the fact that when a patient is cured he does not need to do anything consciously in order to stay cured, although the treatment can always be continued with benefit, since even supernormal vision can be improved.

CHAPTER XIV

IMAGINATION AS AN AID TO VISION

WE see very largely with the mind, and only partly with the eyes. The phenomena of vision depend upon the mind's interpretation of the impression upon the retina. What we see is not that impression, but our own interpretation of it. Our impressions of size, color, form and location can be demonstrated to depend upon the interpretation by the mind of the retinal picture. The moon looks smaller at the zenith than it does at the horizon, though the optical angle is the same and the impression on the retina may be the same, because at the horizon the mind unconsciously compares the picture with the pictures of surrounding objects, while at the zenith there is nothing to compare it with. The figure of a man on a high building, or on the topmast of a vessel, looks small to the landsman; but to the sailor it appears to be of ordinary size, because he is accustomed to seeing the human figure in such positions.

Persons with normal vision use their memory, or imagination, as an aid to sight; and when the sight is imperfect it can be demonstrated, not only that the eye itself is at fault, but that the memory and imagination are impaired, so that the mind adds imperfections to the imperfect retinal image. No two persons with normal sight will get the same visual impressions from the same object; for their interpretations of the retinal picture will differ as much as their individualities differ, and when the sight is imperfect the interpretation is far more variable. It reflects, in fact, the loss of mental control which is responsible for the error of refraction. When the eye is out of focus, in short, the mind is also out of focus.

According to the accepted view most of the abnormalities of vision produced when there is an error of refraction in the eye are sufficiently accounted for by the existence of that error. Some are supposed to be due to diseases of the brain or retina. Multiple images are attributed to astigmatism, though only two can be legitimately accounted for in this way, while some patients state that they see half a dozen or more, and many persons with astigmatism do not see any. It can easily be demonstrated, however, that the inaccuracy of the focus accounts for only a small part of these results; and since they can all be corrected in a few seconds through the correction, by relaxation, of the error of refraction, it is evident that they cannot be due to any organic disease.

If we compare the picture on the glass screen of the camera when the camera is out of focus with the visual impressions of the mind when the eye is out of focus, there will be found to be a great difference between them. When the camera is out of focus it turns black into grey, and blurs the outlines of the picture; but it produces these results uniformly and constantly. On the screen of the camera an imperfect picture of a black letter would be equally imperfect in all parts, and the same adjustment of the focus would always produce the same picture. But when the eye is out of focus the imperfect picture which the patient imagines that he sees is always changing, whether the focus changes or not. There will be more grey on one part than on another, and both the shade and the position of the grey may vary within wide limits in a very short space of time. One part of the letter may appear grey and the rest black. Certain outlines may be seen better than others, the vertical lines, perhaps, appearing black and the diagonal grey, and vice versa. Again, the black may be changed into brown, yellow, green, or even red, transmutations impossible to the camera. Or there may be spots of color, or of black, on the grey, or on the white openings. There may also be spots of white, or of color, on the black.

When the camera is out of focus the picture which it produces of any object is always slightly larger than the image produced when the focus is correct; but when the eye is out of focus the picture which the mind sees may be either larger or smaller than it normally would be. To one patient the big C at ten feet appeared smaller than at either twenty feet or four inches. To some it appears larger than it actually is at twenty feet, and to others it seems smaller.

When the human eye is out of focus the form of the objects regarded by the patient frequently appears to be distorted, while their location may also appear to change. The image may be doubled, tripled, or still further multiplied, and while one object, or part of an object may be multiplied other objects or parts of objects in the field of vision may remain single. The location of these multiple images is sometimes constant and at others subject to continual change. Nothing like this could happen when the camera is out of focus.

If two cameras are out of focus to the same degree, they will take two imperfect pictures exactly alike. If two eyes are out of focus to the same degree, similar impressions will be made upon the retina of each; but the impressions made upon the mind may be totally unlike, whether the eyes belong to the same person or to different persons. If the normal eye looks at an object through glasses that change its refraction, the greyness and blurring produced are uniform and constant; but when the eye has an error of refraction equivalent to that produced by the glasses, these phenomena are non-uniform and variable.

It is fundamental that the patient should understand that these aberrations of vision—which are treated more fully in a later chapter—are illusions, and not due to a fault of the eyes. When he knows that a thing is an illusion he is less likely to see it again. When he becomes convinced that what he sees is imaginary it helps to bring the imagination under control; and since a perfect imagination is impossible without perfect relaxation, a perfect imagination not only corrects the false interpretation of the retinal image, but corrects the error of refraction.

Imagination is closely allied to memory, although distinct from it. Imagination depends upon the memory, because a thing can be imagined only as well as it can be remembered. You cannot imagine a sunset unless you have seen one; and if you attempt to imagine a blue sun, which you have never seen, you will become myopic, as indicated by simultaneous retinoscopy. Neither imagination nor memory can be perfect unless the mind is perfectly relaxed. Therefore when the imagination and memory are perfect, the sight is perfect. Imagination, memory and sight are, in fact, coincident. When one is perfect, all are perfect, and when one is imperfect, all are imperfect. If you imagine a letter perfectly, you will see the letter and other letters in its neighborhood will come out more distinctly, because it is impossible for you to relax and imagine you see a perfect letter and at the same time strain and actually see an imperfect one. If you imagine a perfect period on the bottom of a letter, you will see the letter perfectly, because you cannot take the mental picture of a perfect period and put it on an imperfect letter. It is possible, however, as pointed out in the preceding chapter, for sight to be unconscious. In some cases patients may imagine the period perfectly, as demonstrated by the retinoscope, without being conscious of seeing the letter; and it is often some time before they are able to be conscious of it without losing the period.

When one treats patients who are willing to believe that the letters can be imagined, and who are content to imagine without trying to see, or compare what they see with what they imagine, which always brings back the strain, very remarkable results are sometimes obtained by the aid of the imagination. Some patients at once become able to read all the letters on the bottom line of the test card after they become able to imagine that they see one letter perfectly black and distinct. The majority, however, are so distracted by what they see when their vision has been improved by their imagination that they lose the latter. It is one thing to be able to imagine perfect sight of a letter, and another to be able to see the letter and other letters without losing control of the imagination.

In myopia the following method is often successful:

First look at a letter at the point at which it is seen best. Then close the eyes and remember it. Repeat until the memory is almost as good as the sight at the near-point. With the test card at a distance of twenty feet, look at a blank surface a foot or more to one side of it, and again remember the letter. Do the same at six inches and at three inches. At the last point note the appearance of the letters on the card—that is, in the eccentric field. If the memory is still perfect, they will appear to be a dim black, not grey, and those nearest the point of fixation will appear blacker than those more distant. Gradually reduce the distance between the point of fixation and the letter until able to look straight at it and imagine that it is seen as well as it is remembered. Occasionally it is well during the practice to close and cover the eyes and remember the letter, or a period, perfectly black. The rest and mental control gained in this way are a help in gaining control when one looks at the test card.

Patients who succeed with this method are not conscious while imagining a perfect letter, of seeing, at the same time, an imperfect one, and are not distracted when their vision is improved by their imagination. Many patients can remember perfectly with their eyes closed, or when they are looking at a place where they cannot see the letter; but just as soon as they look at it they begin to strain and lose control of their memory. Therefore, as the imagination depends upon the memory, they cannot imagine that they see the letter. In such cases it has been my custom to proceed somewhat in the manner described in the preceding chapter. I begin by saying to the patient:

"Can you imagine a black period on the bottom of this letter, and at the same time, while imagining the period perfectly, are you able to imagine that you see the letter?

Sometimes they are able to do this, but usually they are not. In that case they are asked to imagine part of the letter, usually the bottom. When they have become able to imagine this part straight, curved, or open, as the case may be, they become able to imagine the sides and top, while still holding the period on the bottom. But even after they have done this, they may still not be able to imagine the whole letter without losing the period. One may have to coax them along by bringing the card up a little closer, then moving it farther away; for when looking at a surface where there is anything to see, the imagination improves in proportion as one approaches the point where the sight is best, because at that point the eyes are most relaxed. When there is nothing particular to see, the distance makes no difference, because no effort is being made to see.

To encourage patients to imagine they see the letter it seems helpful to keep saying to them over and over again:

"Of course you do not see the letter. I am not asking you to see it. I am just asking you to imagine that you see it perfectly black and perfectly distinct."

When patients become able to see a known letter by the aid of their imagination, they become able to apply the same method to an unknown letter; for just as soon as any part of a letter, such as an area equal to a period, can be imagined to be perfectly black, the whole letter is seen to be black, although the visual perception of this fact may not, at first, last long enough for the patient to become conscious of it.

In trying to distinguish unknown letters, the patient discovers that it is impossible to imagine perfectly unless one imagines the truth; for if a letter, or any part of a letter, is imagined to be other than it is, the mental picture is foggy and inconstant, just like a letter which is seen imperfectly.

The ways in which the imagination can be interfered with are very numerous. There is one way of imagining perfectly and an infinite number of ways of imagining imperfectly. The right way is easy. The mental picture of the thing imagined comes as quick as thought, and can be held more or less continuously. The wrong way is difficult. The picture comes slowly, and is both variable and discontinuous. This can be demonstrated to the patient by asking him first to imagine or remember a black letter as perfectly as possible with the eyes closed, and then to imagine the same letter imperfectly. The first he can usually do easily; but it will be found very difficult to imagine a black letter with clear outlines to be grey, with fuzzy edges and clouded openings, and impossible to form a mental picture of it that will remain constant for an appreciable length of time. The letter will vary in color, shape and location in the visual field, precisely as a letter does when it is seen imperfectly; and just as the strain of imperfect sight produces discomfort and pain, the effort to imagine imperfectly will sometimes produce pain. The more nearly perfect the mental picture of the letter, on the contrary, the more easily and quickly it comes and the more constant it is.

Some very dramatic cures have been effected by means of the imagination. One patient, a physician, who had worn glasses for forty years and who could not without them see the big C at twenty feet, was cured in fifteen minutes simply by imagining that he saw the letters black. When asked to describe the big C with unaided vision he said it looked grey to him, and that the opening was obscured by a grey cloud to such an extent that he had to guess that it had an opening. He was told that the letter was black, perfectly black, and that the opening was perfectly white, with no grey cloud; and the card was brought close to him so that he could see that this was so. When he again regarded the letter at the distance, he remembered its blackness so vividly that he was able to imagine that he saw it just as black as he had seen it at the near-point, with the opening perfectly white; and therefore he saw the letter on the card perfectly black and distinct. In the same way he became able to read the seventy line; and so he went down the card, until in about five minutes he became able to read at twenty feet the line which the normal eye is supposed to read at ten feet. Next diamond type was given to him to read. The letters appeared grey to him, and he could not read them. His attention was called to the fact that the letters were really black, and immediately he imagined that he saw them black and became able to read them at ten inches.

The explanation of this remarkable occurrence is simply relaxation. All the nerves of the patient's body were relaxed when he imagined that he saw the letters black, and when he became conscious of seeing the letters on the card, he still retained control of his imagination. Therefore he did not begin to strain again, and actually saw the letters as black as he imagined them.

The patient not only had no relapse, but continued to improve. About a year later I visited him in his office and asked him how he was getting on. He replied that his sight was perfect, both for distance and the near-point. He could see the motor cars on the other side of the Hudson River and the people in them, and he could read the names of boats on the river which other people could make out only with a telescope. At the same time he had no difficulty in reading the newspapers, and to prove the latter part of this statement, he picked up a newspaper and read a few sentences aloud. I was astonished, and asked him how he did it.

"I did what you told me to do," he said.

"What did I tell you to do?" I asked.

"You told me to read the Snellen test card every day, which I have done, and to read fine print every day in a dim light, which I have also done."

Another patient, who had a high degree of myopia complicated with atrophy of the optic nerve, and who had been discouraged by many physicians, was benefited so wonderfully and rapidly by the aid of his imagination that one day while in the office he lost control of himself completely, and raising a test card which he held in his hand, he threw it across the room.

"It is too good to be true," he exclaimed; "I cannot believe it. The possibility of being cured and the fear of disappointment are more than I can stand."

He was calmed down with some difficulty and encouraged to continue. Later he became able to read the small letters on the test card with normal vision. He was then given fine print to read. When he looked at the diamond type, he at once said that it was impossible for him to read it. However, he was told to follow the same procedure that had benefited his distance sight. That is, he was to imagine a period on one part of the small letters while holding the type at six inches. After testing his memory of the period a number of times, he became able to imagine he saw a period perfectly black on one of the small letters. Then he lost control of his nerves again, and on being asked, "What is the trouble?" he said:

"I am beginning to read the fine print, and I am so overwhelmed that I lose my self-control."

In another case, that of a woman with high myopia complicated with incipient cataract, the vision improved in a few days from 3/200 to 20/50. Instead of going gradually down the card, a jump was made from the fifty line to the ten line. The card was brought up close to her, and she was asked to look at the letter O at three inches, the distance at which she saw it best, to imagine that she saw a period on the bottom of it and that the bottom was the blackest part. When she was able to do this at the near-point, the distance was gradually increased until she became able to see the O at three feet. Then I placed the card at ten feet and she exclaimed:

"Oh, doctor, it is impossible! The letter is too small. It is too great a thing for me to do. Let me try a larger letter first."

Nevertheless she became able in fifteen minutes to read the small O on the ten line at twenty-feet.

CHAPTER XV

SHIFTING AND SWINGING

WHEN the eye with normal vision regards a letter either at the near-point or at the distance, the letter may appear to pulsate, or to move in various directions, from side to side, up and down, or obliquely. When it looks from one letter to another on the Snellen test card, or from one side of a letter to another, not only the letter, but the whole line of letters and the whole card, may appear to move from side to side. This apparent movement is due to the shifting of the eye, and is always in a direction contrary to its movement. If one looks at the top of a letter, the letter is below the line of vision, and, therefore, appears to move downward. If one looks at the bottom, the letter is above the line of vision and appears to move upward. If one looks to the left of the letter, it is to the right of the line of vision and appears to move to the right. If one looks to the right, it is to the left of the line of vision and appears to move to the left.

Persons with normal vision are rarely conscious of this illusion, and may have difficulty in demonstrating it; but in every case that has come under my observation they have always become able, in a longer or shorter time, to do so. When the sight is imperfect the letters may remain stationary, or even move in the same direction as the eye.

It is impossible for the eye to fix a point longer than a fraction of a second. If it tries to do so, it begins to strain and the vision is lowered. This can readily be demonstrated by trying to hold one part of a letter for an appreciable length of time. No matter how good the sight, it will begin to blur, or even disappear, very quickly, and sometimes the effort to hold it will produce pain. In the case of a few exceptional people a point may appear to be held for a considerable length of time; the subjects themselves may think that they are holding it; but this is only because the eye shifts unconsciously, the movements being so rapid that objects seem to be seen all alike simultaneously.

The shifting of the eye with normal vision is usually not conspicuous, but by direct examination with the ophthalmoscope it can always be demonstrated. If one eye is examined with this instrument while the other is regarding a small area straight ahead, the eye being examined, which follows the movements of the other, is seen to move in various directions, from side to side, up and down in an orbit which is usually variable. If the vision is normal these movements are extremely rapid and unaccompanied by any appearance of effort. The shifting of the eye with imperfect sight, on the contrary, is slower, its excursions are wider, and the movements are jerky and made with apparent effort.

It can also be demonstrated that the eye is capable of shifting with a rapidity which the ophthalmoscope cannot measure. The normal eye can read fourteen letters on the bottom line of a Snellen test card, at a distance of ten or fifteen feet, in a dim light, so rapidly that they seem to be seen all at once. Yet it can be demonstrated that in order to recognize the letters under these conditions it is necessary to make about four shifts to each letter. At the near-point, even though one part of the letter is seen best, the rest may be seen well enough to be recognized; but at the distance it is impossible to recognize the letters unless one shifts from the top to the bottom and from side to side. One must also shift from one letter to another, making about seventy shifts in a fraction of a second.

A line of small letters on the Snellen test card may be less than a foot long by a quarter of an inch in height; and if it requires seventy shifts to a fraction of a second to see it apparently all at once, it must require many thousands to see an area of the size of the screen of a moving picture, with all its detail of people, animals, houses, or trees, while to see sixteen such areas to a second, as is done in viewing moving pictures, must require a rapidity of shifting that can scarcely be realized. Yet it is admitted that the present rate of taking and projecting moving pictures is too slow. The results would be more satisfactory, authorities say, if the rate were raised to twenty, twenty-two, or twenty-four a second.

The human eye and mind are not only capable of this rapidity of action, and that without effort or strain, but it is only when the eye is able to shift thus rapidly that eye and mind are at rest, and the efficiency of both at their maximum. It is true that every motion of the eye produces an error of refraction; but when the movement is short, this is very slight, and usually the shifts are so rapid that the error does not last long enough to be detected by the retinoscope, its existence being demonstrable only by reducing the rapidity of the movements to less than four or five a second. The period during which the eye is at rest is much longer than that during which an error of refraction is produced. Hence, when the eye shifts normally no error of refraction is manifest. The more rapid the unconscious shifting of the eye, the better the vision; but if one tries to be conscious of a too rapid shift, a strain will be produced.

Perfect sight is impossible without continual shifting, and such shifting is a striking illustration of the mental control necessary for normal vision. It requires perfect mental control to think of thousands of things in a fraction of a second; and each point of fixation has to be thought of separately, because it is impossible to think of two things, or of two parts of one thing, perfectly at the same time. The eye with imperfect sight tries to accomplish the impossible by looking fixedly at one point for an appreciable length of time; that is, by staring. When it looks at a strange letter and does not see it, it keeps on looking at it in an effort to see it better. Such efforts always fail, and are an important factor in the production of imperfect sight.

One of the best methods of improving the sight, therefore, is to imitate consciously the unconscious shifting of normal vision and to realize the apparent motion produced by such shifting. Whether one has imperfect or normal sight, conscious shifting and swinging are a great help and advantage to the eye; for not only may imperfect sight be improved in this way, but normal sight may be improved also. When the sight is imperfect, shifting, if done properly, rests the eye as much as palming, and always lessens or corrects the error of refraction.

The eye with normal sight never attempts to hold a point more than a fraction of a second, and when it shifts, as explained in the chapter on "Central Fixation," it always sees the previous point of fixation worse. When it ceases to shift rapidly and to see the point shifted from worse, the sight ceases to be normal, the swing being either prevented or lengthened, or (occasionally) reversed. These facts are the keynote of the treatment by shifting.

In order to see the previous point of fixation worse, the eye with imperfect sight has to look farther away from it than does the eye with normal sight. If it shifts only a quarter of an inch, for instance, it may see the previous point of fixation as well as or better than before; and instead of being rested by such a shift, its strain will be increased, there will be no swing, and the vision will be lowered. At a couple of inches it may be able to let go of the first point; and if neither point is held more than a fraction of a second, it will be rested by such a shift and the illusion of swinging may be produced. The shorter the shift the greater the benefit; but even a very long shift—as much as three feet or more — is a help to those who cannot accomplish a shorter one. When the patient is capable of a short shift, on the contrary, the long shift lowers the vision. The swing is an evidence that the shifting is being done properly, and when it occurs the vision is always improved. It is possible to shift without improvement; but it is impossible to produce the illusion of a swing without improvement, and when this can be done with a long shift, the movement can gradually be shortened until the patient can shift from the top to the bottom of the smallest letter, on the Snellen test card or elsewhere, and maintain the swing. Later he may become able to be conscious of the swinging of the letters without conscious shifting.

No matter how imperfect the sight, it is always possible to shift and produce a swing, so long as the previous point of fixation is seen worse. Even diplopia and polyopia[1] do not prevent swinging with some improvement of vision. Usually the eye with imperfect vision is able to shift from one side of the card to the other, or from a point above the card to a point below it, and observe that in the first case the card appears to move from side to side, while in the second it appears to move up and down.

When patients are suffering from high degrees of eccentric fixation, it may be necessary, in order to help them to see worse when they shift, to use some of the methods described in the chapter on "Central Fixation." Usually, however, patients who cannot see worse when they shift at the distance can do it readily at the near-point, as the sight is best at that point, not only in myopia, but often in hypermetropia as well. When the swing can be produced at the near point, the distance can be gradually increased until the same thing can be done at twenty feet.

After resting the eyes by closing or palming, shifting and swinging are often more successful. By this method of alternately resting the eyes and then shifting, persons with very imperfect sight have sometimes obtained a temporary or permanent cure in a few weeks.

Shifting may be done slowly or rapidly, according to the state of the vision. At the beginning the patient will be likely to strain if he shifts too rapidly; and then the point shifted from will not be seen worse, and there will be no swing. As improvement is made, the speed can be increased. It is usually impossible, however, to realize the swing if the shifting is more rapid than two or three times a second.

---

[1] Double and multiple vision.

A mental picture of a letter can, as a rule, be made to swing precisely as can a letter on the test card. Occasionally one meets a patient with whom the reverse is true; but for most patients the mental swing is easier at first than visual swinging; and when they become able to swing in this way, it becomes easier for them to swing the letters on the test card. By alternating mental with visual swinging and shifting, rapid progress is sometimes made. As relaxation becomes more perfect, the mental swing can be shortened, until it becomes possible to conceive and swing a letter the size of a period in a newspaper. This is easier, when it can be done, than swinging a larger letter, and many patients have derived great benefit from it.

All persons, no matter how great their error of refraction, when they shift and swing successfully, correct it partially or completely, as demonstrated by the retinoscope, for at least a fraction of a second. This time may be so short that the patient is not conscious of improved vision; but it is possible for him to imagine it, and then it becomes easier to maintain the relaxation long enough to be conscious of the improved sight. For instance, the patient, after looking away from the card, may look back to the big C, and for a fraction of a second the error of refraction may be lessened or corrected, as demonstrated by the retinoscope. Yet he may not be conscious of improved vision. By imagining that the C is seen better, however, the moment of relaxation may be sufficiently prolonged to be realized.

When swinging, either mental or visual, is successful, the patient may become conscious of a feeling of relaxation which is manifested as a sensation of universal swinging. This sensation communicates itself to any object of which the patient is conscious. The motion may be imagined in any part of the body to which the attention is directed. It may be communicated to the chair in which the patient is sitting, or to any object in the room, or elsewhere, which is remembered. The building, the city, the whole world, in fact, may appear to be swinging. When the patient becomes conscious of this universal swinging, he loses the memory of the object with which it started; but so long as he is able to maintain the movement in a direction contrary to the original movement of the eyes, or the movement imagined by the mind, relaxation is maintained. If the direction is changed, however, strain results. To imagine the universal swing with the eyes closed is easy, and some patients soon become able to do it with the eyes open. Later the feeling of relaxation which accompanies the swing may be realized without consciousness of the latter; but the swing can always be produced when the patient thinks of it.

There is but one cause of failure to produce a swing, and that is strain. Some people try to make the letters swing by effort. Such efforts always fail. The eyes and mind do not swing the letters, they swing of themselves. The eye can shift voluntarily. This is a muscular act resulting from a motor impulse. But the Swing comes of its own accord when the shifting is normal. It does not produce relaxation, but is an evidence of it; and while of no value in itself is, like the period, very valuable as an indication that relaxation is being maintained.

The following methods of shifting have been found useful in various cases:

No. 1—

(a) Regard a letter.

(b) Shift to a letter on the same line far enough away so that the first is seen worse.

(c) Look back at No. 1 and see No. 2 worse.

(d) Look at the letters alternately for a few seconds, seeing worse the one not regarded.

When successful, both letters improve and appear to move from side to side in a direction opposite to the movement of the eye.

No. 2—

(a) Look at a large letter.

(b) Look at a smaller one a long distance away from it. The large one is then seen worse.

(c) Look back and see it better.

(d) Repeat half a dozen times.

When successful, both letters improve, and the card appears to move up and down.

No. 3—

Shifting by the above methods enables the patient to see one letter on a line better than the other letters, and, usually, to distinguish it in flashes. In order to see the letter continuously it is necessary to become able to shift from the top to the bottom, or from the bottom to the top, seeing worse the part not directly regarded, and producing the illusion of a vertical swing.

(a) Look at a point far enough above the top of the letter to see the bottom, or the whole letter worse.

(b) Look at a point far enough below the bottom to see the top, or the whole letter, worse.

(c) Repeat half a dozen times.

If successful, the letter will appear to move up and down, and the vision will improve. The shift can then be shortened until it becomes possible to shift between the top and the bottom of the letter and maintain the swing. The letter is now seen continuously. If the method fails, rest the eyes, palm, and try again.

One may also practice by shifting from one side of the letter to a point beyond the other side, or from one corner to a point beyond the other corner.

No. 4—

    (a) Regard a letter at the distance at which it is seen best. In myopia this will be at the near-point, a foot or less from the face. Shift from the top to the bottom until able to see each worse alternately, when the letter will appear blacker than before, and an illusion of swinging will be produced.

    (b) Now close the eyes, and shift from the top to the bottom of the letter mentally.

    (c) Regard a blank wall with the eyes open, and do the same. Compare the ability to shift and swing mentally with the ability to do the same visually at the near-point.

    (d) Then regard the letter at the distance, and shift from the top to the bottom. If successful, the letter will improve, and an illusion of swinging will be produced.

No. 5—

Some patients, particularly children, are able to see better when one points to the letters. In other cases

this is a distraction. When the method is found successful one can proceed as follows:

> (a)   Place the tip of the finger three or four inches
> below the letter. Let the patient regard the
> letter, and shift to the tip of the finger, see-
> ing the letter worse.

> (b)   Reduce the distance between the finger and
> the letter, first to two or three inches, then
> to one or two, and finally to half an inch,
> proceeding each time as in (a).

If successful, the patient will become able to look
from the top to the bottom of the letter, seeing each
worse alternately, and producing the illusion of swinging. It will then be possible to see the letter continuously.

No. 6—

When the vision is imperfect it often happens that,
when the patient looks at a small letter, some of the
larger letters on the upper lines, or the big C at the top,
look blacker than the letter regarded. This makes it
impossible to see the smaller letters perfectly. To correct this eccentric fixation regard the letter which is seen
best, and shift to the smaller letter. If successful, the
small letter, after a few movements, will appear blacker
than the larger one. If not successful after a few trials,
rest the eyes by closing and palming, and try again.
One may also shift from the large letter to a point some
distance below the small letter, gradually approaching
the latter as the vision improves.

No. 7—

Shifting from a card at three or five feet to one at ten
or twenty feet often proves helpful, as the unconscious

memory of the letter seen at the near-point helps to bring out the one at the distance.

Different people will find these various methods of shifting more or less satisfactory. If any method does not succeed, it should be abandoned after one or two trials and something else tried. It is a mistake to continue the practice of any method which does not yield prompt results. The cause of the failure is strain, and it does no good to continue the strain.

When it is not possible to practice with the Snellen test card, other objects may be utilized. One can shift, for instance, from one window of a distant building to another, or from one part of a window to another part of the same window, from one auto to another, or from one part of an auto to another part, producing, in each case, the illusion that the objects are moving in a direction contrary to the movement of the eye. When talking to people, one can shift from one person to another, or from one part of the face to another part. When reading a book, or newspaper, one can shift consciously from one word or letter to another, or from one part of a letter to another.

Shifting and swinging, as they give the patient something definite to do, are often more successful than other methods of obtaining relaxation, and in some cases remarkable results have been obtained simply by demonstrating to the patient that staring lowers the vision and shifting improves it. One patient, a girl of sixteen with progressive myopia, obtained very prompt relief by shifting. She came to the office wearing a pair of glasses tinted a pale yellow, with shades at the sides; and in spite of this protection she was so annoyed by the light that her eyes were almost closed, and she had great difficulty in finding her way about the room. Her vision without glasses was 3/200. All reading had been forbidden, playing the piano from the notes was not allowed, and she had been obliged to give up the idea of going to college. The sensitiveness to light was relieved in a few minutes by focussing the light of the sun upon the upper part of the eyeball when she looked far down, by means of a burning glass (see Chapter XVII). The patient was then seated before a Snellen test card and directed to look away from it, rest her eyes, and then look at the big C. For a fraction of a second her vision was improved, and by frequent demonstrations she was made to realize that any effort to see the letters always lowered the vision. By alternately looking away, and then looking back at the letters for a fraction of a second, her vision improved so rapidly that in the course of half an hour it was almost normal for the distance. Then diamond type was given her to read. The attempt to read it at once brought on a severe pain. She was directed to proceed as she had in reading the Snellen test card; and in a few minutes, by alternately looking away and then looking at the first letter of each word in turn, she became able to read without fatigue, discomfort, or pain. She left the office without her glasses, and was able to see her way without difficulty. Other patients have been benefited as promptly by this simple method.

CHAPTER XVI

THE ILLUSIONS OF IMPERFECT AND
OF NORMAL EYESIGHT

PERSONS with imperfect sight always have illusions of vision; so do persons with normal sight. But while the illusions of normal sight are an evidence of relaxation, the illusions of imperfect sight are an evidence of strain. Some persons with errors of refraction have few illusions, others have many; because the strain which causes the error of refraction is not the same strain that is responsible for the illusions.

The illusions of imperfect sight may relate to the color, size, location and form of the objects regarded. They may include appearances of things that have no existence at all, and various other curious and interesting manifestations.

ILLUSIONS OF COLOR

When a patient regards a black letter and believes it to be grey, yellow, brown, blue, or green, he is suffering from an illusion of color. This phenomenon differs from color-blindness. The color-blind person is unable to differentiate between different colors, usually blue and green, and his inability to do so is constant. The person suffering from an illusion of color does not see the false colors constantly or uniformly. When he looks at the Snellen test card the black letters may appear to him at one time to be grey; but at another moment they may appear to be a shade of yellow, blue, or brown. Some patients always see the black letters red; to others, they appear red only occasionally. Although the letters are all of the same color, some may see the large letters black and the small ones yellow or blue. Usually the large letters are seen darker than the small ones, whatever color they appear to be. Often different colors appear in the same letter, part of it seeming to be black, perhaps, and the rest grey or some other color. Spots of black, or of color, may appear on the white; and spots of white, or of color, on the black.

ILLUSIONS OF SIZE

Large letters may appear small, or small letters large. One letter may appear to be of normal size, while another of the same size and at the same distance may appear larger or smaller than normal. Or a letter may appear to be of normal size at the near-point and at the distance, and only half that size at the middle distance. When a person can judge the size of a letter correctly at all distances up to twenty feet his vision is normal. If the size appears different to him at different distances, he is suffering from an illusion of size. At great distances the judgment of size is always imperfect, because the sight at such distances is imperfect, even though perfect at ordinary distances. The stars appear to be dots, because the eye does not possess perfect vision for objects at such distances. A candle seen half a mile away appears smaller than at the near-point; but seen through a telescope giving perfect vision at that distance it will be the same as at the near-point. With improved vision the ability to judge size improves.

The correction of an error of refraction by glasses seldom enables the patient to judge size as correctly as the normal eye does, and the ability to do this may differ very greatly in persons having the same error of refraction. A person with ten diopters of myopia corrected by glasses may (rarely) be able to judge the sizes of objects correctly. Another person, with the same degree of myopia and the same glasses, may see them only one-half or one-third their normal size. This indicates that errors of refraction have very little to do with incorrect perceptions of size.

ILLUSIONS OF FORM

Round letters may appear square or triangular; straight letters may appear curved; letters of regular form may appear very irregular; a round letter may appear to have a checker-board or a cross in the center. In short, an infinite variety of changing forms may be seen. Illumination, distance and environment are all factors in this form of imperfect sight. Many persons can see the form of a letter correctly when other letters are covered, but when the other letters are visible they cannot see it. The indication of the position of a letter by a pointer helps some people to see it. Others are so disturbed by the pointer that they cannot see the letter so well.

ILLUSIONS OF NUMBER

Multiple images are frequently seen by persons with imperfect sight, either with both eyes together, with each eye separately, or with only one eye. The manner in which these multiple images make their appearance is sometimes very curious. For instance, a patient with presbyopia read the word HAS normally with both eyes. The word PHONES he read correctly with the left eye;

but when he read it with the right eye he saw the letter P double, the imaginary image being a little distance to the left of the real one. The left eye, while it had normal vision for the word PHONES, multiplied the shaft of a pin when this object was in a vertical position (the head remaining single), and multiplied the head when the position was changed to the horizontal (the shaft then remaining single). When the point of the pin was placed below a very small letter, the point was sometimes doubled while the letter remained single. No error of refraction can account for these phenomena. They are tricks of the mind only. The ways in which multiple images are arranged are endless. They are sometimes placed vertically, sometimes horizontally or obliquely, and sometimes in circles, triangles and other geometrical forms. Their number, too, may vary from two to three, four, or more. They may be stationary, or may change their position more or less rapidly. They also show an infinite variety of color, including a white even whiter than that of the background.

ILLUSIONS OF LOCATION

A period following a letter on the same horizontal level as the bottom of the letter may appear to change its position in a great variety of curious ways. Its distance from the letter may vary. It may even appear on the other side of the letter. It may also appear above or below the line. Some persons see letters arranged in irregular order. In the case of the word AND, for instance, the D may occupy the place of the N, or the first letter may change places with the last. All these things are mental illusions. The letters sometimes appear to be farther off than they really are. The small letters, twenty feet distant, may appear to be a mile away. Patients troubled by illusions of distance sometimes ask if the position of the card has not been changed.

ILLUSIONS OF NON-EXISTENT OBJECTS

When the eye has imperfect sight the mind not only distorts what the eye sees, but it imagines that it sees things that do not exist. Among illusions of this sort are the floating specks which so often appear before the eyes when the sight is imperfect, and even when it is ordinarily very good. These specks are known scientifically as "muscæ volitantes," or "flying flies," and although they are of no real importance, being symptoms of nothing except mental strain, they have attracted so much attention, and usually cause so much alarm to the patient, that they will be discussed at length in another chapter.

ILLUSIONS OF COMPLEMENTARY COLORS

When the sight is imperfect, the subject, on looking away from a black, white, or brightly colored object, and closing the eyes, often imagines for a few seconds that he sees the object in a complementary, or approximately complementary, color. If the object is black upon a white background, a white object upon a black background will be seen. If the object is red, it may be seen as blue; and if it is blue, it may appear to be red. These illusions, which are known as "after-images," may also be seen, though less commonly, with the eyes open, upon any background at which the subject happens to look, and are often so vivid that they appear to be real.

ILLUSIONS OF THE COLOR OF THE SUN

Persons with normal sight see the sun white, the whitest white there is; but when the sight is imperfect it may appear to be any color in the spectrum—red, blue, green, purple, yellow, etc. In fact, it has even been described by persons with imperfect vision as totally black. The setting sun commonly appears to be red, because of atmospheric conditions; but in many cases these conditions are not such as to change the color, and while this still appears to be red to persons with imperfect vision, to persons with normal vision it appears to be white. When the redness of a red sun is an illusion, and not due to atmosphere conditions, its image on the ground glass of a camera will be white, not red, and the rays focussed with a burning glass will also be white. The same is true of a red moon.

BLIND SPOTS AFTER LOOKING AT THE SUN

After looking at the sun, most people see black or colored spots which may last from a few minutes to a year or longer, but are never permanent. These spots are also illusions, and are not due, as is commonly supposed, to any organic change in the eye. Even the total blindness which sometimes results, temporarily, from looking at the sun, is only an illusion.

ILLUSIONS OF TWINKLING STARS

The idea that the stars should twinkle has been embodied in song and story, and is generally accepted as part of the natural order of things; but it can be demonstrated that this appearance is simply an illusion of the mind.

CAUSE OF THE ILLUSIONS OF IMPERFECT SIGHT

All the illusions of imperfect sight are the result of a strain of the mind, and when the mind is disturbed for any reason, illusions of all kinds are very likely to occur. This strain is not only different from the strain that produces the error of refraction, but it can be demonstrated that for each and every one of these illusions there is a different kind of strain. Alterations of color do not necessarily affect the size or form of objects, or produce any other illusion, and it is possible to see the color of a letter, or of a part of a letter, perfectly, without recognizing the letter. To change black letters into blue, or yellow, or another color, requires a subconscious strain to remember or imagine the colors concerned, while to alter the form requires a subconscious strain to see the form in question. With a little practice anyone can learn to produce illusions of form and color by straining consciously in the same way that one strains unconsciously; and whenever illusions are produced in this way it will be found that eccentric fixation and an error of refraction have also been produced.

The strain which produces polyopia is different again from the strain which produces illusions of color, size and form. After a few attempts most patients easily learn to produce polyopia at will. Staring or squinting, if the strain is great enough, will usually make one see double. By looking above a light, or a letter, and then trying to see it as well as when directly regarded, one can produce an illusion of several lights, or letters, arranged vertically. If the strain is great enough, there may be as many as a dozen of them. By looking to the side of the light or letter, or looking away obliquely at any angle, the images can be made to arrange themselves horizontally, or obliquely at any angle.

To see objects in the wrong location, as when the first letter of a word occupies the place of the last, requires an ingenuity of eccentric fixation and an education of the imagination which is unusual.

The black or colored spots seen after looking at the sun, and the strange colors which the sun sometimes seems to assume, are also the result of the mental strain. When one becomes able to look at the orb of day without strain, these phenomena immediately disappear.

After-images have been attributed to fatigue of the retina, which is supposed to have been so overstimulated by a certain color that it can no longer perceive it, and therefore seeks relief in the hue which is complementary to this color. If it gets tired looking at the black C on the Snellen test card, for instance, it is supposed to seek relief by seeing the C white. This explanation of the phenomenon is very ingenious but scarcely plausible. The eyes cannot see when they are closed; and if they appear to see under these conditions, it is obvious that the subject is suffering from a mental illusion with which the retina has nothing to do. Neither can they see what does not exist; and if they appear to see a white C on a green wall where there is no such object, it is obvious again that the subject is suffering from a mental illusion. The after-image indicates, in fact, simply a loss of mental control, and occurs when there is an error of refraction, because this condition also is due to a loss of mental control. Anyone can produce an after-image at will by trying to see the big C all alike—that is, under a strain;

but one can look at it indefinitely by central fixation without any such result.

While persons with imperfect sight usually see the stars twinkle, they do not necessarily do so. Therefore it is evident that the strain which causes the twinkling is different from that which causes the error of refraction. If one can look at a star without trying to see it, it does not twinkle; and when the illusion of twinkling has been produced, one can usually stop it by "swinging" the star. On the other hand, one can start the planets, or even the moon, to twinkling, if one strains sufficiently to see them.

ILLUSIONS OF NORMAL SIGHT

The illusions of normal sight include all the phenomena of central fixation. When the eye with normal sight looks at a letter on the Snellen test card, it sees the point fixed best, and everything else in the field of vision appears less distinct. As a matter of fact, the whole letter and all the letters may be perfectly black and distinct, and the impression that one letter is blacker than the others, or that one part of a letter is blacker than the rest, is an illusion. The normal eye, however, may shift so rapidly that it appears to see a whole line of small letters all alike simultaneously. As a matter of fact there is, of course, no such picture on the retina. Each letter has not only been seen separately, but it has been demonstrated in the chapter on "Shifting and Swinging" that if the letters are seen at a distance of fifteen or twenty feet, they could not be recognized unless about four shifts were made on each letter. To produce the impression of a simultaneous picture of fourteen letters, therefore, some sixty or seventy pictures, each with some one point more distinct than the rest, must have been produced upon the retina. The idea that the letters are seen all alike simultaneously is therefore, an illusion. Here we have two different kinds of illusions. In the first case the impression made upon the brain is in accordance with the picture on the retina, but not in accordance with the fact. In the second the mental impression is in accordance with the fact, but not with the pictures upon the retina.

The normal eye usually sees the background of a letter whiter than it really is. In looking at the letters on the Snellen test card it sees white streaks at the margins of the letters, and in reading fine print it sees between the lines and the letters, and in the openings of the letters, a white more intense than the reality. Persons who cannot read fine print may see this illusion, but less clearly. The more clearly it is seen, the better the vision; and if it can be imagined consciously—it is imagined unconsciously when the sight is normal—the vision improves. If the lines of fine type are covered, the streaks between them disappear. When the letters are regarded through a magnifying glass by the eye with normal sight, the illusion is not destroyed, but the intensity of the white and black are lessened. With imperfect sight it may be increased to some extent by this means, but will remain less intense than the white and black seen by the normal eye. The facts demonstrate that perfect sight cannot be obtained with glasses.

The illusions of movement produced by the shifting of the eye and described in detail in the chapter on "Shifting and Swinging" must also be numbered among the illusions of normal sight, and so must the perception of objects in an upright position.   This last is the most curious illusion of all.   No matter what the position of the head, and regardless of the fact that the image on the retina is inverted, we always see things right side up.

CHAPTER XVII

VISION UNDER ADVERSE CONDITIONS
A BENEFIT TO THE EYES

ACCORDING to accepted ideas of ocular hygiene, it is important to protect the eyes from a great variety of influences which are often very difficult to avoid, and to which most people resign themselves with the uneasy sense that they are thereby "ruining their eyesight." Bright lights, artificial lights, dim lights, sudden fluctuations of light, fine print, reading in moving vehicles, reading lying down, etc., have long been considered "bad for the eyes," and libraries of literature have been produced about their supposedly direful effects. These ideas are diametrically opposed to the truth. When the eyes are properly used, vision under adverse conditions not only does not injure them, but is an actual benefit, because a greater degree of relaxation is required to see under such conditions than under more favorable ones. It is true that the conditions in question may at first cause discomfort, even to persons with normal vision; but a careful study of the facts has demonstrated that only persons with imperfect sight suffer seriously from them, and that such persons, if they practice central fixation, quickly become accustomed to them and derive great benefit from them.

Although the eyes were made to react to the light, a very general fear of the effect of this element upon the organs of vision is entertained both by the medical profession and by the laity. Extraordinary precautions are taken in our homes, offices and schools to temper the light, whether natural or artificial, and to insure that it shall not shine directly into the eyes; smoked and amber glasses, eye-shades, broad-brimmed hats and parasols are commonly used to protect the organs of vision from what is considered an excess of light; and when actual disease is present, it is no uncommon thing for patients to be kept for weeks, months and years in dark rooms, or with bandages over their eyes.

The evidence on which this universal fear of the light has been based is of the slightest. In the voluminous literature of the subject one finds such a lack of information that in 1910 Dr. J. Herbert Parsons of the Royal Ophthalmic Hospital of London, addressing a meeting of the Ophthalmological Section of the American Medical Association, felt justified in saying that ophthalmologists, if they were honest with themselves, "must confess to a lamentable ignorance of the conditions which render bright light deleterious to the eyes."[1] Since then, Verhoeff and Bell have reported[2] an exhaustive series of experiments carried on at the Pathological Laboratory of the Massachusetts Charitable Eye and Ear Infirmary, which indicate that the danger of injury to the eye from light radiation as such has been "very greatly exaggerated." That brilliant sources of light sometimes produce unpleasant temporary symptoms cannot, of course, be denied; but as regards definite pathological effects, or permanent impairment of vision from exposure to light alone, Drs. Verhoeff and Bell were unable to find, either clinically or experimentally, anything of a positive nature.

[1] Jour. Am. Med. Assn., Dec. 10, 1910, p. 2028.
[2] Proc. Am. Acad. Arts and Sciences. 1916, Vol. 51, No. 13.

As for danger from the heat effects of light, they consider this to be "ruled out of consideration by the immediate discomfort produced by excessive heat." They conclude, in short, that "the eye in the process of evolution has acquired the ability to take care of itself under extreme conditions of illumination to a degree hitherto deemed highly improbable." In their experiments, the eyes of rabbits, monkeys and human beings were flooded for an hour or more with light of extreme intensity, without any sign of permanent injury, the resulting scotomata[1] disappearing within a few hours. Commercial illuminants were found to be entirely free of danger under any ordinary conditions of their use. It was even found impossible to damage the retina with any artificial illuminant, except by exposures and intensities enormously greater than any likely to occur outside the laboratory. In one case an animal succumbed to heat after an exposure of an hour and a half to a 750-watt nitrogen lamp at twenty centimeters—about eight inches; but in a second experiment, in which it was well protected from the heat, there was no damage to the eye whatever after an exposure of two hours. As for the ultra-violet part of the spectrum, to which exaggerated importance has been attached by many recent writers, the situation was found to be much the same as with respect to the rest of the spectrum; that is, "while under conceivable or realizable conditions of over-exposure, injury may be done to the external eye, yet under all practicable conditions found in actual use of artificial sources of light for illumination, the ultra-violet part of the spectrum may be left out as a possible source of injury."

The results of these experiments are in complete ac-

---

[1] Blind areas.

cord with my own observations as to the effect of strong
light upon the eyes. In my experience such light has
never been permanently injurious. Persons with normal
sight have been able to look at the sun for an indefinite
length of time, even an hour or longer, without any
discomfort or loss of vision. Immediately afterward
they were able to read the Snellen test card with improved vision, their sight having become better than
what is ordinarily considered normal. Some persons with
normal sight do suffer discomfort and loss of vision when
they look at the sun; but in such cases the retinoscope always indicates an error of refraction, showing that this
condition is due, not to the light, but to strain. In exceptional cases, persons with defective sight have been able
to look at the sun, or have thought that they have looked
at it, without discomfort and without loss of vision; but,
as a rule, the strain in such eyes is enormously increased
and the vision decidedly lowered by sun-gazing, as manifested by inability to read the Snellen test card. Blind
areas (scotomata) may develop in various parts of the
field—two or three or more. The sun, instead of appearing perfectly white, may appear to be slate-colored, yellow, red, blue, or even totally black. After looking away
from the sun, patches of color of various kinds and sizes
may be seen, continuing a variable length of time, from
a few seconds to a few minutes, hours, or even months.
In fact, one patient was troubled in this way for a year
or more after looking at the sun for a few seconds. Even
total blindness lasting a few hours has been produced.
Organic changes may also be produced. Inflammation,
redness of the conjunctiva, cloudiness of the lens and of
the aqueous and vitreous humors, congestion and cloudiness of the retina, optic nerve and choroid, have all re-

sulted from sun-gazing. These effects, however, are always temporary. The scotomata, the strange colors, even the total blindness, as explained in the preceding chapter, are only mental illusions. No matter how much the sight may have been impaired by sun-gazing, or how long the impairment may have lasted, a return to normal

Fig. 46.—Woman With Normal Vision Looking Directly at the Sun. Note That the Eyes are Wide Open and That There Is No Sign of Discomfort.

has always occurred; while prompt relief of all the symptoms mentioned has always followed the relief of eye-strain, showing that the conditions are the result, not of the light, but of the strain. Some persons who have believed their eyes to have been permanently injured by the sun have been promptly cured by central fixation, indicating that their blindness had been simply functional.

By persistence in looking at the sun, a person with normal sight soon becomes able to do so without any loss of vision; but persons with imperfect sight usually find it impossible to accustom themselves to such a strong light until their vision has been improved by other means. One has to be very careful in recommending sun-gazing to persons with imperfect sight; because although no permanent harm can result from it, great temporary discomfort may be produced, with no permanent benefit. In some rare cases, however, complete cures have been effected by this means alone.

In one of these cases, the sensitiveness of the patient, even to ordinary daylight, was so great that an eminent specialist had felt justified in putting a black bandage over one eye and covering the other with a smoked glass so dark as to be nearly opaque. She was kept in this condition of almost total blindness for two years without any improvement. Other treatment extending over some months also failed to produce satisfactory results. She was then advised to look directly at the sun. The immediate result was total blindness, which lasted several hours; but next day the vision was not only restored to its former condition, but was improved. The sun-gazing was repeated, and each time the blindness lasted for a shorter period. At the end of a week the patient was able to look directly at the sun without discomfort, and her vision, which had been 20/200 without glasses and 20/70 with them, had improved to 20/10, twice the accepted standard for normal vision.

Patients of this class have also been greatly benefited by focussing the rays of the sun directly upon their eyes, marked relief being often obtained in a few minutes.

Like the sun, a strong electric light may also lower the vision temporarily, but never does any permanent harm.

In those exceptional cases in which the patient can become accustomed to the light, it is beneficial. After looking at a strong electric light some patients have been able to read the Snellen test card better.

Fig. 47. Woman Aged 37, Child Aged 4, Both Looking Directly at Sun Without Discomfort

It is not light but darkness that is dangerous to the eye. Prolonged exclusion from the light always lowers the vision, and may produce serious inflammatory conditions. Among young children living in tenements this is a somewhat frequent cause of ulcers upon the cornea, which ultimately destroy the sight. The children, finding their eyes sensitive to light, bury them in the pillows and thus shut out the light entirely. The universal fear of reading or doing fine work in a dim light is, however, unfounded. So long as the light is sufficient so that one can see without discomfort, this practice is not only harmless, but may be beneficial.

Sudden contrasts of light are supposed to be particularly harmful to the eye. The theory on which this idea is based is summed up as follows by Fletcher B. Dresslar, specialist in school hygiene and sanitation of the United States Bureau of Education:

"The muscles of the iris are automatic in their movements, but rather slow. Sudden contrasts of strong light and weak illumination are painful and likewise harmful to the retina. For example, if the eye, adjusted to a dim light, is suddenly turned toward a brilliantly lighted object, the retina will receive too much light and will be shocked before the muscles controlling the iris can react to shut out the superabundance of light. If contrasts are not strong, but frequently made, that is, if the eye is called upon to function where frequent adjustments in this way are necessary, the muscles controlling the iris become fatigued, respond more slowly and less perfectly. As a result, eyestrain in the ciliary muscles is produced and the retina is over-stimulated. This is one cause of headaches and tired eyes."[1]

There is no evidence whatever to support these statements. Sudden fluctuations of light undoubtedly cause discomfort to many persons, but, far from being injurious, I have found them, in all cases observed, to be actually beneficial. The pupil of the normal eye, when it has normal sight, does not change appreciably under

---

[1] School Hygiene, Brief Course Series in Education, edited by Monroe, 1916, p. 240.

Fig. 48. Focussing the Rays of the Sun Upon the Eye of a
Patient by Means of a Burning Glass

the influence of changes of illumination; and persons with normal vision are not inconvenienced by such changes. I have seen a patient look directly at the sun after coming from an imperfectly lighted room, and then, returning to the room, immediately pick up a newspaper and read it. When the eye has imperfect sight, the pupil usually contracts in the light and expands in the dark, but it has been observed to contract to the size of a pinhole in the dark. Whether the contraction takes place under the influence of light or of darkness, the cause is the same, namely, strain. Persons with imperfect sight suffer great inconvenience, resulting in lowered vision, from changes in the intensity of the light; but the lowered vision is always temporary, and if the eye is persistently exposed to these conditions, the sight is benefited. Such practices as reading alternately in a bright and a dim light, or going from a dark room to a well-lighted one, and vice versa, are to be recommended. Even such rapid and violent fluctuations of light as those involved in the production of the moving picture are, in the long run, beneficial to all eyes. I always advise patients under treatment for the cure of defective vision to go to the movies frequently and practice central fixation. They soon become accustomed to the flickering light, and afterward other light and reflections cause less annoyance.

Reading is supposed to be one of the necessary evils of civilization; but it is believed that by avoiding fine print, and taking care to read only under certain favorable conditions, its deleterious influences can be minimized. Extensive investigations as to the effect of various styles of print on the eyesight of school children have been made, and detailed rules have been laid down as to the size of the print, its shading, the distance of the letters from each other, the spaces between the lines, the length of the lines, etc. As regards the effects of different sorts of type on the human eye in general and those of children in particular, Dr. A. G. Young, in his much quoted report[1] to the Maine State Board of Health makes the following interesting observations:

Pearl, as the printers call it, is unfit for any eyes, yet the piles of Bibles and Testaments annually printed in it tempt many eyes to self-destruction.

Agate is the type in which a boy, to the writer's knowledge, undertook to read the Bible through. His outraged eyes broke down with asthenopia before he went far and could be used but little for school work the next two years.

Nonpareil is used in some papers and magazines for children, but, to spare the eyes, all such should, and do, go on the list of forbidden reading matter in those homes where the danger of such print is understood.

Minion is read by the healthy, normal young eye without appreciable difficulty, but even to the sound eye the danger of strain is so great that all books and magazines for children printed from it should be banished from the home and school.

Brevier is much used in newspapers, but is too small for magazines or books for young folks.

Bourgeois is much used in magazines, but should be used in only those school books to which a brief reference is made.

Long Primer is suitable for school readers for the higher and intermediate grades, and for text books generally.

Small Pica is still a more luxurious type, used in the North American Review and the Forum.

Pica is a good type for books for small children.

Great Primer should be used for the first reading book.

---

[1] Seventh Annual Report to the Maine State Board of Health, by the secretary, Dr. A. G. Young, 1891, p. 193.

All this is directly contrary to my own experience. Children might be bored by books in excessively small print; but I have never seen any reason for supposing that their eyes or any other eyes, would be harmed by such type. On the contrary, the reading of fine print, when it can be done without discomfort, has invariably proved to be beneficial, and the dimmer the light in which it can be read, and the closer to the eyes it can be held, the greater the benefit. By this means severe pain in the eyes has been relieved in a few minutes or even instantly. The reason is that fine print cannot be read in a dim light and close to the eyes unless the eyes are relaxed, whereas large print can be read in a good light and at ordinary reading distance although the eyes may be under a strain. When fine print can be read under adverse conditions, the reading of ordinary print under ordinary conditions is vastly improved. In myopia it may be a benefit to strain to see fine print, because myopia is always lessened when there is a strain to see near objects, and this has sometimes counteracted the tendency to strain in looking at distant objects, which is always associated with the production of myopia. Even straining to see print so fine that it cannot be read is a benefit to some myopes.

Persons who wish to preserve their eyesight are frequently warned not to read in moving vehicles; but since under modern conditions of life many persons have to spend a large part of their time in moving vehicles, and many of them have no other time to read, it is useless to expect that they will ever discontinue the practice. Fortunately the theory of its injuriousness is not borne out by the facts. When the object regarded is moved more or less rapidly, strain and lowered vision are, at

Seven Truths of Normal Sight

1. Normal Sight can always be demonstrated in the normal eye, but only under favorable conditions.
2. Central Fixation: The letter or part of the letter regarded is always seen best.
3. Shifting: The point regarded changes rapidly and continuously.
4. Swinging: When the shifting is slow, the letters appear to move from side to side, or in other directions with a pendulum-like motion.
5. Memory is perfect. The color and background of the letters or other objects seen, are remembered perfectly, instantaneously and continuously.
6. Imagination is good. One may even see the white part of letters whiter than it really is, while the black is not altered by distance, illumination, size, or form, of the letters.
7. Rest or relaxation of the eye and mind is perfect and can always be demonstrated.

When one of these seven fundamentals is perfect, all are perfect.

Fig. 49.   Specimen of Diamond Type

Many patients have been greatly benefited by reading type of this size.

Fig. 50.   Photographic Type Reduction

Patients who can read photographic type reductions are instantly relieved of pain and discomfort when they do so, and those who cannot read such type may be benefited simply by looking at it.

first, always produced; but this is always temporary, and ultimately the vision is improved by the practice.

There is probably no visual habit against which we have been more persistently warned than that of reading in a recumbent posture. Many plausible reasons have been adduced for its supposed injuriousness; but so delightful is the practice that few, probably, have ever been deterred from it by fear of the consequences. It is gratifying to be able to state, therefore, that I have found these consequences to be benefical rather than injurious. As in the case of the use of the eyes under other difficult conditions, it is a good thing to be able to read lying down, and the ability to do it improves with practice. In an upright position, with a good light coming over the left shoulder, one can read with the eyes under a considerable degree of strain; but in a recumbent posture, with the light and the angle of the page to the eye unfavorable, one cannot read unless one relaxes. Anyone who can read lying down without discomfort is not likely to have any difficulty in reading under ordinary conditions.

The fact is that vision under difficult conditions is good mental training. The mind may be disturbed at first by the unfavorable environment; but after it has become accustomed to such environments, the mental control, and, consequently, the eyesight are improved. To advise against using the eyes under unfavorable conditions is like telling a person who has been in bed for a few weeks and finds it difficult to walk to refrain from such exercise. Of course, discretion must be used in both cases. The convalescent must not at once try to run a Marathon, nor must the person with defective vision attempt, without some preparation, to outstare the sun at noonday. But just as the invalid may gradually increase his strength until the Marathon has no terrors for him, so may the eye with defective sight be educated until all the rules with which we have so long allowed ourselves to be harassed in the name of "eye hygiene" may be disregarded, not only with safety but with benefit.

CHAPTER XVIII

OPTIMUMS AND PESSIMUMS

IN nearly all cases of imperfect sight due to errors of refraction there is some object, or objects, which can be regarded with normal vision. Such objects I have called "optimums." On the other hand, there are some objects which persons with normal eyes and ordinarily normal sight always see imperfectly, an error of refraction being produced when they are regarded, as demonstrated by the retinoscope. Such objects I have called "pessimums." An object becomes an optimum, or a pessimum, according to the effect it produces upon the mind, and in some cases this effect is easily accounted for.

For many children their mother's face is an optimum, and the face of a stranger a pessimum. A dressmaker was always able to thread a No. 10 needle with a fine thread of silk without glasses, although she had to put on glasses to sew on buttons, because she could not see the holes. She was a teacher of dressmaking, and thought the children stupid because they could not tell the difference between two different shades of black. She could match colors without comparing the samples. Yet she could not see a black line in a photographic copy of the Bible which was no finer than a thread of silk, and she could not remember a black period. An employee in a cooperage factory, who had been engaged for years in picking out defective barrels as they went rapidly past him on an inclined plane, was able to continue his work

198

after his sight for most other objects had become very defective, while persons with much better sight for the Snellen test card were unable to detect the defective barrels. The familiarity of these various objects made it possible for the subjects to look at them without strain—that is, without trying to see them. Therefore the barrels were to the cooper optimums; while the needle's eye and the colors of silk and fabrics were optimums to the dressmaker. Unfamiliar objects, on the contrary, are always pessimums, as pointed out in the chapter on "The Variability of the Refraction of the Eye."

In other cases there is no accounting for the idiosyncrasy of the mind which makes one object a pessimum and another an optimum. It is also impossible to account for the fact that an object may be an optimum for one eye and not for the other, or an optimum at one time and at one distance and not at others. Among these unaccountable optimums one often finds a particular letter on the Snellen test card. One patient, for instance, was able to see the letter K on the forty, fifteen and ten lines, but could see none of the other letters on these lines, although most patients would see some of them, on account of the simplicity of their outlines, better than they would such a letter as K.

Pessimums may be as curious and unaccountable as optimums. The letter V is so simple in its outlines that many people can see it when they cannot see others on the same line. Yet some people are unable to distinguish it at any distance, although able to read other letters in the same word, or on the same line of the Snellen test card. Some people again will not only be unable to recognize the letter V in a word, but also to read any word that contains it, the pessimum lowering their sight not only for itself but for other objects. Some letters, or objects, become pessimums only in particular situations. A letter, for instance, may be a pessimum when located at the end or at the beginning of a line or sentence, and not in other places. When the attention of the patient is called to the fact that a letter seen in one location ought logically to be seen equally well in others, the letter often ceases to be a pessimum in any situation.

A pessimum, like an optimum, may be lost and later become manifest. It may vary according to the light and distance. An object which is a pessimum in a moderate light may not be so when the light is increased or diminished. A pessimum at twenty feet may not be one at two feet, or thirty feet, and an object which is a pessimum when directly regarded may be seen with normal vision in the eccentric field.

For most people the Snellen test card is a pessimum. If you can see the Snellen test card with normal vision, you can see almost anything else in the world. Patients who cannot see the letters on the Snellen test card can often see other objects of the same size and at the same distance with normal sight. When letters which are seen imperfectly, or even letters which cannot be seen at all, or which the patient is not conscious of seeing are regarded, the error of refraction is increased. The patient may regard a blank white card without any error of refraction; but if he regards the lower part of a Snellen test card, which appears to him to be just as blank as the blank card, an error of refraction can always be demonstrated, and if the visible letters of the card are covered, the result is the same. The pessimum may, in short, be letters or objects which the patient is not conscious of seeing. This phenomenon is very common. When the card is seen in the eccentric field it may have the effect of lowering the vision for the point directly regarded. For instance, a patient may regard an area of green wallpaper at the distance, and see the color as well as at the near-point; but if a Snellen test card on which the letters are either seen imperfectly, or not seen at all, is placed in the neighborhood of the area being regarded, the retinoscope may indicate an error of refraction. When the vision improves, the number of letters on the card which are pessimums diminishes and the number of optimums increases, until the whole card becomes an optimum.

A pessimum, like an optimum, is a manifestation of the mind. It is something associated with a strain to see, just as an optimum is something which has no such association. It is not caused by the error of refraction, but always produces an error of refraction; and when the strain has been relieved it ceases to be a pessimum and becomes an optimum.

CHAPTER XIX

THE RELIEF OF PAIN AND OTHER SYMPTOMS BY THE AID OF THE MEMORY

MANY years ago patients who had been cured of imperfect sight by treatment without glasses quite often told me that after their vision had become perfect they were always relieved of pain, not only in the eyes and head, but in other parts of the body, even when the pain was apparently caused by some organic disease, or by an injury. The relief in many cases was so striking that I investigated some thousands of cases and found it to be a fact that persons with perfect sight, or the memory of perfect sight—that is, of something perfectly seen—do not suffer pain in any part of the body, while by a strain or effort to see I have produced pain in various parts of the body.

By perfect sight is not meant, necessarily, the perfect visual perception of words, letters, or objects, of a more or less complicated form. To see perfectly the color alone is sufficient, and the easiest color to see perfectly is black. But perfect sight is never continuous, careful scientific tests having shown that it is seldom maintained for more than a few minutes and usually not so long. For practical purposes in the relief of pain, therefore, the memory is more satisfactory than sight.

When black is remembered perfectly a temporary, if not a permanent, relief of pain always results. The skin may be pricked with a sharp instrument without causing discomfort. The lobe of the ear may be pinched be-

tween the nails of the thumb and first finger, and no pain
will be felt. At the same time the sense of touch becomes
more acute. The senses of taste, smell and hearing are
also improved, while the efficiency of the mind is increased. The ability to distinguish different temperatures
is increased, but one does not suffer from heat or cold.
Organic conditions may not be changed; but all of the
functional symptoms, such as fever, weakness, and shock,
which these conditions cause, are relieved. Patients who
have learned to remember black under all circumstances
no longer dread to visit the dentist. When they remember a period the drill causes them no pain, and they are
not annoyed even by the extraction of teeth. It is possible to perform surgical operations without anaesthetics
when the patient is able to remember black perfectly.
The following are only a few of many equally striking
cases which might be given of the relief or prevention of
pain by this means:

A patient suffered from ulceration of the eyeball, oc-
curring at different times and resulting in the formation
of holes through which the fluids in the interior escaped.
These openings had to be closed by surgical operations.
At first these operations were performed under the influence of cocaine; but the progressive disease of the eye
caused so much congestion that complete anaesthesia was
no longer attainable by the use of this drug, and ether
and chloroform were employed. As so many operations
were needed, it became desirable to get along, if possible,
without anaesthetics, and the patient's success in relieving pain by the memory of black suggested that she might
also be able to prevent the pain of operations in the same
way. Her ability to do this was tested by touching her
eyeball lightly with a blunt probe. At first she forgot the

black as soon as the probe touched her eye, but later she became able to remember it. The operation was then successfully performed; the patient not only felt no pain,

Fig. 51. Operating Without Anaesthetics

The patient suffered from ulceration of the eyeball resulting in the formation of holes through which the fluids of the interior escaped. These holes had to be closed by surgical operations, and fourteen of these operations were performed without anaesthetics, because the patient was able to prevent pain by the memory of a black period.

but her self-control was better than when cocaine had been used. Later fourteen more operations were performed under the same conditions, the patient not only suffering no pain, but, what was more remarkable, feeling no pain or soreness afterward. The patient stated that if she had been operated upon by a stranger she would probably have been so nervous that she would not have been able to remember the black; but later she was treated by a strange dentist, who made two extractions and did some other work, all without causing her any discomfort, because she was able to remember the period perfectly.

A man who had been extremely nervous in the dentist's chair, and had had four extractions made under gas, surprised his dentist, after having learned the effect of the memory of a period in relieving pain, by having a tooth extracted without cocaine, gas, or chloroform. The dentist complimented him on his nerve and looked incredulous when the patient said he had felt no pain at all. In a second case, that of a woman, the dentist removed the nerve from three teeth without causing the patient any pain.

A boy of fourteen came to the eye clinic of the Harlem Hospital, New York, with a foreign body deeply embedded in his cornea. It caused him much pain, and his mother stated that a number of physicians had been unable to remove it, because the child was so nervous that he could not keep still long enough, although cocaine had been used quite freely. The boy was told to look at a black object, close and cover his eyes, and think of the black object until he saw black. He was soon able to do this, and the pain in his eye was relieved. He was next taught to remember the black with his eyes open. The foreign body was then removed from the cornea. The operation was one of much difficulty and required considerable time, but the boy felt no pain. While it was in progress he was asked if he was still remembering black.

"You bet I am," he replied.

In the same hospital a surgeon from the accident ward visited the eye clinic with a friend suffering from pain in his eyes and head. The patient was benefited very quickly by relaxation methods. The surgeon said it was unusual, and spoke slightingly of my methods. I challenged him to bring me a patient with pain that I could not relieve in five minutes.

"All right," he said. "I want you to understand that I am from Missouri."

He returned soon with a woman who had been suffering from severe pains in her head for several years. She had been operated upon a number of times, and had been under the care of the hospital for many months.

"You cannot help the pain in this patient's head," said the surgeon, "because she has a brain tumor."

I doubted the existence of a brain tumor, but I said: "Brain tumor or no brain tumor, my assistant will stop the pain in five minutes."

He took out his watch, opened it, looked at the time, and told my assistant to go ahead. The patient was directed to look at a large black letter, note its blackness, then to cover her closed eyes with the palms of her hands, shutting out all the light, and to remember the blackness of the letter until she saw everything black. In less than three minutes she said:

"I now see everything perfectly black. I feel no pain in my head. I am completely relieved, and I thank you very much."

The surgeon looked bewildered, and left the room without a word.

Fig. 52. Neuralgia Relieved by Palming and the Memory of Black

While the visitor was explaining to her sceptical hostess the method of relieving pain by palming and the memory of black, another member of the family, who was suffering from trigeminal neuralgia, came in, and having heard what was being said, immediately put it into practice and was cured. The hostess later developed severe pain in her head and eyes, and did not obtain any relief until she also practiced palming and the memory of black.

To prevent a relapse, the patient was advised to palm six times a day or oftener. The pain did not return, and she came to the clinic some weeks later to express her gratitude.

Not only does the memory of perfect sight relieve pain and the symptoms of disease, but in some cases it produces manifest relief of the causes of these symptoms. Coughs, colds, hay fever, rheumatism and glaucoma are among the conditions that have been relieved in this way.

A patient under treatment for imperfect sight from a high degree of mixed astigmatism one day came to the office with a severe cold. She coughed continually, and there was a profuse discharge from both eyes and nose. There was some fever, with a severe pain in the eyes and head, and the patient was unable to breathe through her nose because of the inflammatory swelling. Palming was successful in half an hour, when the pain and discharge ceased, the nose opened, and the breathing and temperature became normal. The benefit was permanent—a very unusual thing after one treatment.

A boy of four with whooping-cough was always relieved by covering his eyes and remembering black. The relapses became less frequent, and in a few weeks he had completely recovered.

A man who suffered every summer from attacks of hay fever, beginning in June and lasting throughout the season was completely relieved by palming for half an hour; and after three years there had been no relapse.

A man of sixty-five who had been under treatment for rheumatism for six months without improvement obtained temporary relief by palming, and by the time his vision had become normal the relief of the rheumatism was complete.

In many cases of glaucoma not only the pain, but the tension which is often associated with the pain, has been completely relieved by palming. In some cases permanent relief of the tension has followed one treatment. In others many treatments have been required.

Why the memory of black should have this effect cannot be fully explained, just as the action of many drugs cannot be explained; but it is evident that the body must be less susceptible to disturbances of all kinds when the mind is under control, and only when the mind is under control can black be remembered perfectly. That pain can be produced in any part of the body by the action of the mind is not a new observation; and if the mind can produce pain, it is not surprising that it should also be able to relieve pain and the conditions which produce it. This, doubtless, is the explanation of some of the remarkable cures reported by Faith Curists and Christian Scientists. Whatever the explanation, however, the facts have been attested by numerous proofs, and are of the greatest practical value.

With a little training, anyone with good sight can be taught to remember black perfectly with the eyes closed and covered, and with a little more training anyone can learn to do it with the eyes open. When one is suffering extreme pain, however, the control of the memory may be difficult, and the assistance of someone who understands the method may be necessary. With such assistance it is seldom or never impossible.

CHAPTER XX

PRESBYOPIA: ITS CAUSE AND CURE

AMONG people living under civilized conditions the accommodative power of the eye gradually declines, in most cases, until at the age of sixty or seventy it appears to have been entirely lost, the subject being absolutely dependent upon his glasses for vision at the near-point. As to whether the same thing happens among primitive people or people living under primitive conditions, very little information is available. Donders[1] says that the power of accommodation diminishes little, if at all, more rapidly among people who use their eyes much at the near-point than among agriculturists, sailors and others who use them mainly for distant vision; and Roosa and others[2] say the contrary. This is a fact however, that people who cannot read, no matter what their age, will manifest a failure of near vision if asked to look at printed characters, although their sight for familiar objects at the near-point may be perfect. The fact that such persons, at the age of forty-five or fifty, cannot differentiate between printed characters is no warrant, therefore, for the conclusion that their accommodative powers are declining. A young illiterate would do no better, and a young student who can read Roman characters at the near-point without difficulty always develops symptoms of imperfect sight when he attempts to read, for the first time, old English, Greek, or Chinese characters.

---

[1] On the Anomalies of Accommodation and Refraction of the Eye, p. 223.
[2] Roosa: A Clinical Manual of Diseases of the Eye, 1894, p. 537; Oliver: System of Diseases of the Eye, vol. iv, p. 431.

When the accommodative power has declined to the point at which reading and writing become difficult, the patient is said to have "presbyopia," or, more popularly, "old sight"; and the condition is generally accepted, both by the popular and the scientific mind, as one of the unavoidable inconveniences of old age. "Presbyopia," says Donders, "is the normal quality of the normal, emmetropic eye in advanced age,"[1] and similar statements might be multiplied endlessly. De Schweinitz calls the condition "a normal result of growing old";[2] according to Fuchs it is "a physiological process which every eye undergoes";[3] while Roosa speaks of the change as one which "ultimately affects every eye."[4]

The decline of accommodative power with advancing years is commonly attributed to the hardening of the lens, an influence which is believed to be augmented, in later years, by a flattening of this body and a lowering of its refractive index, together with weakness or atrophy of the ciliary muscle; and so regular is the decline, in most cases, that tables have been compiled showing the near-point to be expected at various ages. From these it is said one might almost fit glasses without testing the vision of the subject; or, conversely, one might, from a man's glasses, judge his age within a year or two. The following table is quoted from Jackson's chapter on "The Dioptrics of the Eye," in Norris and Oliver's "System of Diseases of the Eye,"[5] and does not differ materially from the tables given by Fuchs, Donders and Duane. The first

---

[1] On the Anomalies of Accommodation and Refraction of the Eye, p. 210.
[2] Diseases of the Eye, p. 148.
[3] Text-book of Ophthalmology, authorized translation from the twelfth German edition by Duane, 1919, p. 862. Ernst Fuchs (1851-   ). Professor of Ophthalmology at Vienna from 1885 to 1915. His Text-book of Ophthalmology has been translated into many languages.
[4] A Clinical Manual of Diseases of the Eye, p. 535.
[5] Vol. i, p. 504.

column indicates the age; the second, diopters of accommodative power; the third, the near-point for an emmetropic[1] eye, in inches.

Age	Diopters	Inches
10	14	2.81
15	12	3.28
20	10	3.94
25	8.5	4.63
30	7	5.63
35	5.5	7.16
40	4.5	8.75
45	3.5	11.25
50	2.5	15.75
55	1.5	26.25
60	.75	52.49
65	.25	157.48
70	0	0

According to these depressing figures, one must expect at thirty to have lost no less than half of one's original accommodative power, while at forty two-thirds of it would be gone, and at sixty it would be practically non-existent.

There are many people, however, who do not fit this schedule. Many persons at forty can read fine print at four inches, although they ought, according to the table, to have lost that power shortly after twenty. Worse still, there are people who refuse to become presbyopic at all. Oliver Wendell Holmes mentions one of these cases in "The Autocrat of the Breakfast Table."

---

[1] An eye which, when it is at rest, focusses parallel rays upon the retina, is said to be emmetropic or normal.

"There is now living in New York State," he says, "an old gentleman who, perceiving his sight to fail, immediately took to exercising it on the finest print, and in this way fairly bullied Nature out of her foolish habit of taking liberties at five-and-forty, or thereabout. And now this old gentleman performs the most extraordinary feats with his pen, showing that his eyes must be a pair of microscopes. I should be afraid to say how much he writes in the compass of a half-dime—whether the Psalms or the Gospels, or the Psalms and the Gospels, I won't be positive."[1]

There are also people who regain their near vision after having lost it for ten, fifteen, or more years; and there are people who, while presbyopic for some objects, have perfect sight for others. Many dressmakers, for instance, can thread a needle with the naked eye, and with the retinoscope it can be demonstrated that they accurately focus their eyes upon such objects; and yet they cannot read or write without glasses.

So far as I am aware no one but myself has ever observed the last mentioned class of cases, but the others are known to every opththalmologist of any experience. One hears of them at the meetings of ophthalmological societies; they are even reported in the medical journals; but such is the force of authority that when it comes to writing books they are either ignored or explained away, and every new treatise that comes from the press repeats the old superstition that presbyopia is "a normal result of growing old." We have beaten Germany; but the dead hand of German science still oppresses our intellects and prevents us from crediting the plainest evidence of our senses. Some of us are so filled with repugnance for

---

[1] Everyman's Library, 1908, pp. 166-167.

the Hun that we can no longer endure the music of Bach, or the language of Goethe and Schiller; but German ophthalmology is still sacred, and no facts are allowed to cast discredit upon it.

Fortunately for those who feel called upon to defend the old theories, myopia postpones the advent of presbyopia, and a decrease in the size of the pupil, which often takes place in old age, has some effects in facilitating vision at the near-point. Reported cases of persons reading without glasses when over fifty-or fifty-five years of age, therefore, can be easily disposed of by assuming that the subjects must be myopic, or that their pupils are unusually small. If the case comes under actual observation, the matter may not be so simple, because it may be found that the patient, so far from being myopic, is hypermetropic, or emmetropic, and that the pupil is of normal size. There is nothing to do with these cases but to ignore them. Abnormal changes in the form of the lens have also been held responsible for the retention of near vision beyond the prescribed age, or for its restoration after it has been lost, the swelling of the lens in incipient cataract affording a very convenient and plausible explanation for the latter class of cases. In cases of premature presbyopia "accelerated sclerosis"[1] of the lens and weakness of the ciliary muscle have been assumed; and if such cases as the dressmakers who can thread their needles when they can no longer read the newspapers had been observed, no doubt some explanation consistent with the German viewpoint would have been found for them.

The truth about presbyopia is that it is not "a normal result of growing old," being both preventable and cu-

[1] Fuchs: Text-book of Ophthalmology, p. 905.

rable. It is not caused by hardening of the lens, but by a strain to see at the near-point. It has no necessary connection with age, since it occurs, in some cases, as early as ten years, while in others it never occurs at all, although the subject may live far into the so-called presbyopic age. It is true that the lens does harden with advancing years, just as the bones harden and the structure of the skin changes; but since the lens is not a factor in accommodation, this fact is immaterial, and while in some cases the lens may become flatter, or lose some of its refractive power with advancing years, it has been observed to remain perfectly clear and unchanged in shape up to the age of ninety. Since the ciliary muscle is also not a factor in accommodation, its weakness or atrophy can contribute nothing to the decline of accommodative power. Presbyopia is, in fact, simply a form of hypermetropia in which the vision for the near-point is chiefly affected, although the vision for the distance, contrary to what is generally believed, is always lowered also. The difference between the two conditions is not always clear. A person with hypermetropia may or may not read fine print, and a person at the presbyopic age may read it without apparent inconvenience and yet have imperfect sight for the distance. In both conditions the sight at both points is lowered, although the patient may not be aware of it.

It has been shown that when the eyes strain to see at the near-point the focus is always pushed farther away than it was before, in one or all meridians; and by means of simultaneous retinoscopy it can always be demonstrated that when a person with presbyopia tries to read fine print and fails, the focus is always pushed farther away than it was before the attempt was made, indicating that the failure was caused by strain. Even the thought of making such an effort will produce strain, so that the refraction may be changed, and pain, discomfort and fatigue produced, before the fine print is regarded. Furthermore, when a person with presbyopia rests the eyes by closing them, or palming, he always becomes able, for a few moments at least, to read fine print at six inches, again indicating that his previous failure was due, not to any fault of the eyes, but to a strain to see. When the strain is permanently relieved, the presbyopia is permanently cured, and this has happened, not in a few cases, but in many, and at all ages, up to sixty, seventy and eighty.

The first patient that I cured of presbyopia was myself. Having demonstrated by means of experiments on the eyes of animals that the lens is not a factor in accommodation, I knew that presbyopia must be curable, and I realized that I could not look for any very general acceptance of the revolutionary conclusions I had reached so long as I wore glasses myself for a condition supposed to be due to the loss of the accommodative power of the lens. I was then suffering from the maximum degree of presbyopia. I had no accommodative power whatever, and had to have quite an outfit of glasses, because with a glass, for instance, which enabled me to read fine print at thirteen inches, I could not read it either at twelve inches or at fourteen. The retinoscope showed that when I tried to see anything at the near-point without glasses, my eyes were focussed for the distance, and when I tried to see anything at the distance they were focussed for the near-point. My problem, then, was to find some way of reversing this condition and inducing my eyes to focus for the point I wished to see at the moment that I wished to see it. I consulted various eye specialists but my language was to them like that of St. Paul to the Greeks, namely, foolishness. "Your lens is as hard as a stone," they said. "No one can do anything for you." Then I went to a nerve specialist. He used the retinoscope on me, and confirmed my own observations as to the peculiar contrariness of my accommodation; but he had no idea what I could do about it. He would consult some of his colleagues, he said, and asked me to come back in a month, which I did. Then he told me he had come to the conclusion that there was only one man who could cure me, and that was Dr. William H. Bates of New York.

"Why do you say that?" I asked.

"Because you are the only man who seems to know anything about it," he answered.

Thus thrown upon my own resources, I was fortunate enough to find a non-medical gentleman who was willing to do what he could to assist me, the Rev. R. B. B. Foote, of Brooklyn. He kindly used the retinoscope through many long and tedious hours while I studied my own case, and tried to find some way of accommodating when I wanted to read, instead of when I wanted to see something at the distance. One day, while looking at a picture of the Rock of Gibralter which hung on the wall, I noted some black spots on its face. I imagined that these spots were the openings of caves, and that there were people in these caves moving about. When I did this my eyes were focussed for the reading distance. Then I looked at the same picture at the reading distance, still imagining that the spots were caves with people in them. The retinoscope showed that I had accommodated, and I was able to read the lettering beside the picture. I had, in fact, been temporarily cured by the use of my imagination. Later I found that when I imagined the letters black I was able to see them black, and when I saw them black I was able to distinguish their form. My progress after this was not what could be called rapid. It was six months before I could read the newspapers with any kind of comfort, and a year before I obtained my present accommodative range of fourteen inches, from four inches to eighteen; but the experience was extremely valuable, for I had in pronounced form every symptom subsequently observed in other presbyopic patients.

Fortunately for the patients, it has seldom taken me as long to cure other people as it did to cure myself. In some cases a complete and permanent cure was effected in a few minutes. Why, I do not know. I will never be satisfied till I find out. A patient who had worn glasses for presbyopia for about twenty years was cured in less than fifteen minutes by the use of his imagination.

When asked to read diamond type, he said he could not do so, because the letters were grey and looked all alike. I reminded him that the type was printer's ink and that there was nothing blacker than printer's ink. I asked him if he had ever seen printer's ink. He replied that he had. Did he remember how black it was? Yes. Did he believe that these letters were as black as the ink he remembered? He did, and then he read the letters; and because the improvement in his vision was permanent, he said that I had hypnotized him.

In another case a presbyope of ten years' standing was cured just as quickly by the same method. When reminded that the letters which he could not read were black, he replied that he knew they were black, but that they looked grey.

"If you know they are black, and yet see them grey," I said, "you must imagine them grey. Suppose you imagine that they are black. Can you do that?"

"Yes," he said, "I can imagine that they are black"; and then he proceeded to read them.

These extremely quick cures are rare. In nine cases out of ten progress has been much slower, and it has been necessary to resort to all the methods of obtaining relaxation found useful in the treatment of other errors of refraction. In the more difficult cases of presbyopia the patients often suffer from the same illusions of color, size, form and number, when they try to read fine print, as do patients with hypermetropia, astigmatism, and myopia when they try to read the letters on the Snellen test card at the distance. They are unable to remember or imagine, when trying to see at the near-point, even such a simple thing as a small black spot, but can remember it perfectly when they do not try to see. Their sight for the distance is often very imperfect and always below normal, although they may have thought it perfect; and just as in the case of other errors of refraction, improvement of the distant vision improves the vision at the near-point. Regardless, however, of the difficulty of the case and the age of the patient, some improvement has always been obtained, and if the treatment was continued long enough, the patient has been cured.

The idea that presbyopia is a normal result of growing old is responsible for much defective eyesight. When people who have reached the presbyopic age experience difficulty in reading, they are very likely to resort at once to glasses, either with or without professional advice. In some cases such persons may be actually presbyopic; in others the difficulty may be something temporary, which they would have thought little about if they had been younger, and which would have passed away if Nature had been left to herself. But once the glasses are adopted, in the great majority of cases, they produce the condition they were designed to relieve, or, if it already existed, they make it worse, sometimes very rapidly, as every ophthalmologist knows. In a couple of weeks, sometimes, the patient finds, as noted in the chapter on "What Glasses Do to Us," that the large print which he could read without difficulty before he got his glasses, can no longer be read without their aid. In from five to ten years the accommodative power of the eye is usually gone; and if from this point the patient does not go on to cataract, glaucoma, or inflammation of the retina, he may consider himself fortunate. Only occasionally do the eyes refuse to submit to the artificial conditions imposed upon them; but in such cases they may keep up an astonishing struggle against them for long periods. A woman of seventy, who had worn glasses for twenty years, was still able to read diamond type and had good vision for the distance without them. She said the glasses tired her eyes and blurred her vision, but that she had persisted in wearing them, in spite of a continual temptation to throw them off, because she had been told that it was necessary for her to do so.

If persons who find themselves getting presbyopic, or who have arrived at the presbyopic age, would, instead of resorting to glasses, follow the example of the gentleman mentioned by Dr. Holmes, and make a practice of reading the finest print they can find, the idea that the decline of accommodative power is "a normal result of growing old" would soon die a natural death.

CHAPTER XXI

SQUINT AND AMBLYOPIA: THEIR CAUSE

SINCE we have two eyes, it is obvious that in the act of sight two pictures must be formed; and in order that these two pictures shall be fused into one by the mind, it is necessary that there shall be perfect harmony of action between the two organs of vision. In looking at a distant object the two visual axes must be parallel, and in looking at an object at a less distance than infinity, which for practical purposes is less than twenty feet, they must converge to exactly the same degree. The absence of this harmony of action is known as "squint," or "strabismus," and is one of the most distressing of eye defects, not only because of the lowering of vision involved, but because the want of symmetry in the most expressive feature of the face which results from it has a most unpleasant effect upon the personal appearance. The condition is one which has long baffled ophthalmological science. While the theories as to its cause advanced in the text-books seem to fit some cases, they leave others unexplained, and all methods of treatment are admitted to be very uncertain in their results.

The idea that a lack of harmony in the movements of the eye is due to a corresponding lack of harmony in the strength of the muscles that turn them in their sockets seemed such a natural one that this theory was almost universally accepted at one time. Operations based upon it once had a great vogue; but to-day they are advised, by most authorities, only as a last resort. It is true that many persons have been benefited by them; but, at best, the correction of the squint is only approximate, and in many cases the condition has been made worse, while a restoration of binocular vision—the power of fusing the two visual images into one—is scarcely even hoped for.[1]

The muscle theory fitted the facts so badly that when Donders advanced the idea that squint was a condition growing out of refractive errors—hypermetropia being held responsible for the production of convergent and myopia for divergent squint—it was universally accepted. This theory, too, proved unsatisfactory, and now medical opinion is divided between various theories.   Hansen-Grut attributed the condition, in the great majority of cases, to a defect, not of the muscles, but of the nerve supply; and this idea has had many supporters.   Worth and his disciples lay stress on the lack of a so-called fusion faculty, and have recommended the use of prisms, or other measures, to develop it.   Stevens believes that the anomaly results from a wrong shape of the orbit, and as it is impossible to alter this condition, advocates operations for the purpose of neutralizing its influence.

In order to make any of these theories appear consistent it is necessary to explain away a great many troublesome facts.   The uncertain result of operations upon the eye muscles is sufficient to cast suspicion on the theory that the condition is due to any abnormality of the muscles, and many cases of marked paralysis of one or more muscles have been observed in which there was no squint. Relief of paralysis, moreover, may not relieve the squint, nor the relief of the squint the paralysis.   Worth found

---

[1] The result obtained by the operation is, as a rule, simply cosmetic. The sight of the squinting eye is not influenced by the operation, and in only a few instances is even binocular vision restored.—Fuchs: Text-book of Ophthalmology, p. 795.
    The result of even the most successful squint operation, in long-standing strabismus, is merely cosmetic in the vast majority of cases.—Eversbusch: The Diseases of Children, edited by Pfaunder and Schlossman.   English translation by Shaw and La Fetra, second edition, 1912-1914, vol. vii, p. 316.

so many cases which were not benefited by training designed to improve the fusion faculty that he recommended operations on the muscles in such cases; while
Donders, noting that the majority of hypermetropes did
not squint, was obliged to assume that hypermetropia

Fig. 53

No. 1—Reading the Snellen test card with normal vision;
visual axes parallel.

No. 2—The same patient making an effort to see the test
card; myopia and convergent squint of the left eye have been
produced.

did not cause this condition without the aid of co-oper-
ating circumstances.

That the state of the vision is not an important factor
in the production of squint is attested by a multitude of
facts.   It is true, as Donders observed, that squint is
usually associated with errors of refraction; but some
people squint with a very slight error of refraction.   It
is also true that many persons with convergent squint

have hypermetropia; but many others have not. Some persons with convergent squint have myopia. A person may also have convergent squint with one eye normal and one hypermetropic or myopic, or with one eye blind. Usually the vision of the eye that turns in is less than that of the eye which is straight; yet there are cases in which the eye with the poorer vision is straight and the eye with the better vision turned in. With two blind eyes, both eyes may be straight, or one may turn in. With one good eye and one blind eye, both eyes may be straight. The blinder the eye, as a rule, the more marked the squint; but exceptions are frequent, and in rare cases an eye with nearly normal vision may turn in persistently. A squint may disappear and return again, while convergent squint will change into divergent squint and back again. With the same error of refraction, one person will have squint and the other not. A third will squint with a different eye. A fourth will squint first with one eye and then with the other. In a fifth the amount of the squint will vary. One will get well without glasses, or other treatment, and another with these things. These cures may be temporary, or permanent, and the relapses may occur either with or without glasses.

However slight the error of refraction, the vision of many squinting eyes is inferior to that of the straight eye, and for this condition, usually, no apparent or sufficient cause can be found in the constitution of the eye. There is a difference of opinion as to whether this curious defect of vision is the result of the squint, or the squint the result of the defect of vision; but the predominating opinion that it is, at least, aggravated by the squint has been crystallized in the name given to the condition, namely, "amblyopia ex anopsia," literally "dim-sightedness from non-use"—for in order to avoid the annoyance of double vision the mind is believed to suppress the image of the deviating eye. There are, however, many squinting eyes without amblyopia, while such a condition has been found in eyes that have never squinted.

The literature of the subject is full of the impossibility of curing amblyopia, and in popular writings persons having the care of children are urged to have cases of squint treated early, so that the vision of the squinting eye may not be lost. According to Worth, not much improvement can ordinarily be obtained in amblyopic eyes after the age of six, while Fuchs says,[1] "The function of the retina never again becomes perfectly normal, even if the cause of the visual disturbance is done away with." Yet it is well known, as the translator of Fuchs points out in an editorial comment upon the above statement,[2] that if the sight of the good eye is lost at any period of life, the vision of the amblyopic eye will often become normal. Furthermore, an eye may be amblyopic at one time and not at another. When the good eye is covered, a squinting eye may be so amblyopic that it can scarcely distinguish daylight from darkness; but when both eyes are open, the vision of the squinting eye may be found to be as good as that of the straight eye, if not better. In many cases, too, the amblyopia will change from one eye to the other.

Double vision occurs very seldom in squint, and when it does, it often assumes very curious forms. When the eyes turn in the image seen by the right eye should, according to all the laws of optics, be to the right, and the image seen by the left eye to the left. When the

---

[1] Text-book of Ophthalmology, p. 633.
[2] Cases have been reported, some surely authentic, in which an amblyopic squinting eye has acquired good vision, either through correction of the refraction, or because loss of sight in the good eye has compelled the use of the amblyopic eye.—Ibid.

eyes turn out, the opposite should be the case. But often the position of the images is reversed, the image of the right eye in convergent squint being seen to the left and that of the left eye to the right, while in divergent squint the opposite is the case. This condition is known as "paradoxical diplopia." Furthermore, persons with almost normal vision and both eyes perfectly straight may have both kinds of double vision.

All the theories heretofore suggested fail to explain the foregoing facts; but it is a fact that in all cases of squint a strain can be demonstrated, and that the relief of the strain is in all cases followed by the cure of the squint, as well as of the amblyopia and the error of refraction. It is also a fact that all persons with normal eyes can produce squint by a strain to see. It is not a difficult thing to do, and many children derive much amusement from the practice, while it gives their elders unnecessary concern, for fear the temporary squint may become permanent. To produce convergent squint is comparatively easy. Children usually do it by straining to see the end of the nose. The production of divergent squint is more difficult, but with practice persons with normal eyes become able to turn out either eye, or both, at will. They also become able to turn either eye upward and inward, or upward and outward, at any desired angle. Any kind of squint can, in fact, be produced at will by the appropriate kind of strain. Some persons retain the power to produce voluntary squint more or less permanently. Others quickly lose it if they do not keep in practice. There is usually a lowering of the vision when voluntary squint is produced, and accepted methods of measuring the strength of the muscles seem to show deficiencies corresponding to the nature of the squint.

CHAPTER XXII

SQUINT AND AMBLYOPIA: THEIR CURE

THE evidence is conclusive that squint and amblyopia, like errors of refraction, are purely functional troubles; and since they are always relieved by the relief of the strain with which they are associated, it follows that any of the methods which promote relaxation and central fixation may be employed for their cure. As in the case of errors of refraction, the squint disappears and the amblyopia is corrected just as soon as the patient gains sufficient mental control to remember a perfectly black period. In this way both conditions can be temporarily relieved in a few seconds, their permanent cure being a mere matter of making this temporary state permanent.

One of the best ways of gaining mental control in cases of squint is to learn how to increase the squint, or produce other kinds of squint, voluntarily. In the case illustrated, the patient had divergent vertical squint in both eyes. When the left eye was straight the right eye turned out and up, and when the right eye was straight the left eye turned down and out. Both eyes were amblyopic and there was double vision, with the images sometimes on the same side and sometimes on opposite sides. The patient suffered from headaches, and having obtained no relief from glasses, or other methods of treatment, she made up her mind to an operation and consulted Dr. Gudmund J. Gislason, of Grand Forks, N. D., with a view to having one performed. Dr. Gislason, puzzled to find so many muscles apparently

227

at fault, asked my opinion as to which of them should be operated upon. I showed the patient how to make her squint worse, and recommended that Dr. Gislason treat her by eye education without an operation. He did so, and in less than a month the patient had learned to turn both eyes in voluntarily. At first she did this by looking at a pencil held over the bridge of the nose; but later she became able to do it without the pencil, and ultimately she became able to produce every kind of squint at will. The treatment was not pleasant for her, because the production of new kinds of squint, or the making worse of the existing condition, gave her pain; but it effected a complete and permanent cure both of the squint and of the amblyopia. The same method has proved successful with other patients.

Some patients do not know whether they are looking straight at an object or not. These may be helped by watching the deviating eye and directing them to look more nearly in the proper direction. When the deviating eye looks directly at an object, the strain to see is less, and the vision is consequently improved. Covering the good eye with an opaque screen, or with ground glass, encourages a more proper use of the squinting eye, especially if the vision of that eye is imperfect.

Children of six years, or younger, can usually be cured of squint by the use of atropine, a one per cent solution being instilled into one or both eyes twice a day, for many months, a year, or longer. The atropine makes it more difficult for the child to see, and makes the sunlight disagreeable. In order to overcome this handicap it has to relax, and the relaxation cures the squint.

The improvement resulting from eye education in cases of squint and amblyopia is sometimes so rapid as to be almost incredible. The following are a few of many other examples that might be quoted:

A girl of eleven had convergent vertical squint of the left eye. The vision of this eye at the distance was 3/200, while at the near-point it was so imperfect that she was unable to read. The vision of the right eye was normal both for the near-point and the distance. She was wearing glasses when she came to the office—convex 4.00 D. S. combined with convex 0.50 D. C., axis 90, for the right eye; and convex 5.50 D. S. for the left eye—but had obtained no benefit from them. When she looked three feet away from the big C with the left eye, she saw it better than when she looked directly at it; but when asked to count my fingers held three feet away from the card, they so attracted her attention that she was able to see the large letter worse. The fact was impressed upon her that she could see the card better when she looked away from it, or she could see it worse, at will; and she was also asked to note that when she saw it worse her vision improved, and when she saw it better her vision declined. After shifting from the card to a point three feet away from it, and seeing the former worse a few times, her vision improved to 10/200. The ability to shift and see worse improved by practice so rapidly that in less than ten days her vision was normal in both eyes, and in less than two weeks it had improved to 20/10, while diamond type was read with each eye at from three inches to twenty inches. In less than three weeks her vision for the distance was 20/5, by artificial light, and she read photographic type reductions at two inches, the tests being made with both eyes together and with each eye separately. She also read strange test cards as readily as the familiar ones. She

Fig. 54.   Case of Divergent Vertical Squint Cured by
Eye Education

No. 1.—The right eye turns out and up, the left being straight.
No. 2.   The patient learns to look down and out with the
left eye while the right looks straight.

No. 3.—The patient learns to turn both eyes in by looking at
a pencil held over the bridge of the nose.

No. 4.—The patient is permanently cured.

All four pictures were taken within fifteen minutes of each
other, the patient having learned to reproduce the conditions
represented at will.

was advised to continue the treatment at home to prevent a relapse, and at the end of three years none had occurred. During the treatment at the office and practice at home the good eye was covered with an opaque screen, but this was not worn at other times.

A very remarkable case was that of a girl of fourteen who had squinted from childhood. The internal rectus of the right eye had been cut when she was two years old, but still pulled the eye inward. The patient objected to wearing a ground glass over her good eye, because her friends teased her about it and she thought it made her more conspicuous than the squint. One day she lost her glasses in the snow; but her father, who was a man of strong character, immediately provided another pair. Then she announced that she was ill, and couldn't go to school. I told the father that his daughter was hysterical, and simply imagined she was ill to avoid treatment. He insisted that she continue, and as she did not consider herself well enough to come to see me, I called upon her. With the assistance of her father she was made to understand that she would have to continue the treatment until she was cured, and she at once went to work with such energy and intelligence that in half an hour the vision of the squinting and amblyopic eye had improved from 3/200 to 20/30. She also became able to read fine print at twelve inches. She went back to school wearing the ground glass over the good eye; but whenever she wanted to see she looked over the top of it. Her father followed her to school, and insisted that she use the poorer eye instead of the better one. She became convinced that the simplest way out of her troubles would be to follow my instructions, and in less than a week the squint was corrected and she had perfect vision in both eyes. At the beginning of the treatment she could not count her fingers at three feet with the poorer eye, and in three weeks, including all the time that she wasted, she had perfect sight. When told that she was cured her

Fig. 55

No. 1.—Convergent squint of the right eye.

No. 2.—The patient is temporarily cured by the memory of a black period.

main concern seemed to be to know whether she would have to wear the ground glass any more. She was assured that she would not have to do so unless there was a relapse, but there never was any relapse.[1]

---

[1] Bates: L'éducation de l'oeil dans l'amblyopie ex anopsia, Clin. Opht., Dec. 10, 1912.

A girl of eight had had amblyopia and squint since childhood. The vision of the right eye was 10/40, while that of the left was 20/30. Glasses did not improve either eye. The patient was seated twenty feet from a Snellen test card and the right, or poorer eye, was covered with an opaque screen. She was directed to look with her better eye at the large letter on the card and to note its clearness. Next she was told to look at a point three feet to one side of the card, and her attention was called to the fact that she did not then see the large letter so well. The point of fixation was brought closer and closer to the letter, until she appreciated the fact that her vision was lowered when she looked only a few inches to one side of it. When she looked at a small letter she readily recognized that an eccentric fixation of less than an inch lowered the vision.

After she had learned to increase the amblyopia of the better eye, this eye was covered while she was taught how to lower the vision of the other, or poorer eye, by increasing its eccentric fixation. This was accomplished in a few minutes. She was told that the cause of her defective sight was her habit of looking at objects with a part of the retina to one side of the true center of sight. She was advised to see by looking straight at the Snellen card. In less than half an hour the vision of the left eye became normal, while the right improved from 10/40 to 10/10. The cure was complete in two weeks.

The following case was unusually prolonged, because as soon as one eye had been cured, the defect for which it had been treated appeared in the other eye. The patient, a child of ten, had imperfect sight in both eyes, but worse in the right than in the left. The vision of the right eye was restored after some weeks by eye education, when the left eye turned in and became amblyopic. The right eye was then covered, and after a few weeks of eye education the left became normal. The right eye then turned in and the vision became defective. It was necessary to educate the eyes alternately, for about a year, before both became normal at the same time. This patient had congenital paralysis of the external rectus muscle in both eyes, a condition which was apparently not relieved when the squint and amblyopia were cured.

In the following case the patient had an attack of infantile paralysis after her cure, resulting in a relapse, with new and more serious developments, which were, however quickly cured. The patient, a girl of six, seen first on December 11, 1914, had had divergent squint of the left eye for three years, and had worn glasses for two years without benefit—convex 2.50 D. S. for the right eye, and convex 6.00 D. S. combined with convex 1.00 D. C., axis 90, for the left. The vision of the right eye with glasses was 12/15 and of the left 12/200. Atropine was prescribed for the right eye for the purpose of partially blinding it and thus encouraging a more nearly proper use of the squinting eye, and the usual methods of securing relaxation, such as shifting, palming, the exercise of the memory, etc., were used. On January 13, 1915, the vision without glasses had improved to 10/70 for the right eye, and 10/50 for the left. On February 6, the vision of the right eye was 10/40 and of the left 10/30. The eyes were apparently straight, and scientific tests showed that both were used at the same time (binocular single vision). On April 17, after about four months' treatment, the vision of the left eye was normal, and there was binocular single vision at six inches. On May 1 the vision of the left eye was still normal, and whereas at the beginning the patient had been unable to read with it at all, even with glasses, she now read diamond type without glasses at six inches.

On August 16, 1916, the patient had an attack of infantile paralysis which was then epidemic. The sight of both eyes failed, the muscles that turned the eyes in and out were paralyzed, the eyelids twitched, and there was double vision. Various muscles of the head, the left leg and the left arm were also paralzyed. When she left the hospital after five weeks the left eye was turned in, and the vision of both eyes was so poor that she was unable to recognize her mother. Later she developed alternate convergent squint. On November 2 the paralysis in the right eye subsided, and four weeks later that of the left eye began to improve. On November 9 she returned for treatment without any conspicuous squint, but still suffering from double vision, with the images sometimes on the same side and sometimes on opposite sides. On November 23 the eyes were straight and the vision normal.

On July 11, 1918, the eyes were still straight and the vision normal, and there was binocular single vision at six inches. Although atropine had been used in the right eye every day for more than a year, and intermittently for a much longer time, and the pupil was dilated to the maximum, it read fine print without difficulty at six inches, central fixation overcoming the paralyzing effect of the drug. According to the current theory the accommodation should have been completely paralyzed, making near vision quite impossible. The patient also read fine print with the left eye as well as, or better than, with the right eye.

CHAPTER XXIII

FLOATING SPECKS: THEIR CAUSE AND CURE

A VERY common phenomenon of imperfect sight is the one known to medical science as "muscae volitantes" or "flying flies." These floating specks are usually dark or black, but sometimes appear like white bubbles, and in rare cases may assume all the colors of the rainbow. They move somewhat rapidly, usually in curving lines, before the eyes, and always appear to be just beyond the point of fixation. If one tries to look at them directly, they seem to move a little farther away. Hence their name of "flying flies."

The literature of the subject is full of speculations as to the origin of these appearances. Some have attributed them to the presence of floating specks—dead cells or the débris of cells—in the vitreous humor, the transparent substance that fills four-fifths of the eyeball behind the crystalline lens. Similar specks on the surface of the cornea have also been held responsible for them. It has even been surmised that they might be caused by the passage of tears over the cornea. They are so common in myopia that they have been supposed to be one of the symptoms of this condition, although they occur also with other errors of refraction, as well as in eyes otherwise normal. They have been attributed to disturbances of the circulation, the digestion and the kidneys, and because so many insane people have them, have been thought to be an evidence of incipient insanity. The patent-medicine business has thrived upon them, and it would be difficult to estimate the amount of mental torture they have caused, as the following cases illustrate.

A clergyman who was much annoyed by the continual appearance of floating specks before his eyes was told by his eye specialist that they were a symptom of kidney disease, and that in many cases of kidney trouble disease of the retina might be an early symptom. So at regular intervals he went to the specialist to have his eyes examined, and when at length the latter died, he looked around immediately for some one else to make the periodical examination. His family physician directed him to me. I was by no means so well known as his previous ophthalmological adviser, but it happened that I had taught the family physician how to use the ophthalmoscope after others had failed to do so. He thought, therefore, that I must know a lot about the use of the instrument, and what the clergyman particularly wanted was some one capable of making a thorough examination of the interior of his eyes and detecting at once any signs of kidney disease that might make their appearance. So he came to me, and at least four times a year for ten years he continued to come.

Each time I made a very careful examination of his eyes, taking as much time over it as possible, so that he would believe that it was careful; and each time he went away happy because I could find nothing wrong. Once when I was out of town he got a cinder in his eye, and went to another oculist to get it out. When I came back late at night I found him sitting on my doorstep, on the chance that I might return. His story was a pitiable one. The strange doctor had examined his eyes with the ophthalmoscope, and had suggested the possibility of glaucoma, describing the disease as a very treacherous one which might cause him to go suddenly blind and would be agonizingly painful. He emphasized what the patient had previously been told about the danger of kidney disease, suggested that the liver and heart might also be involved, and advised him to have all of these organs carefully examined. I made another examination of his eyes in general and their tension in particular; I had him feel his eyeballs and compare them with my own, so that he might see for himself that they were not becoming hard as a stone; and finally I succeeded in reassuring him. I have no doubt, however, that he went at once to his family physician for an examination of his internal organs.

A man returning from Europe was looking at some white clouds one day when floating specks appeared before his eyes. He consulted the ship's doctor, who told him that the symptom was very serious, and might be the forerunner of blindness. It might also indicate incipient insanity, as well as other nervous or organic diseases. He advised him to consult his family physician and an eye specialist as soon as he landed, which he did. This was twenty-five years ago, but I shall never forget the terrible state of nervousness and terror into which the patient had worked himself by the time he came to me. It was even worse than that of the clergyman, who was always ready to admit that his fears were unreasonable. I examined his eyes very carefully, and found them absolutely normal. The vision was perfect both for the near-point and the distance. The color perception, the fields and the tension were normal; and under a strong magnifying glass I could find no opacities in the vitreous. In short, there were absolutely no symptoms of any disease. I told the patient there was nothing wrong with his eyes, and I also showed him an advertisement of a quack medicine in a newspaper which gave a great deal of space to describing the dreadful things likely to follow the appearance of floating specks before the eyes, unless you began betimes to take the medicine in question at one dollar a bottle. I pointed out that the advertisement, which was appearing in all the big newspapers of the city every day, and probably in other cities, must have cost a lot of money, and must, therefore, be bringing in a lot of money. Evidently there must be a great many people suffering from this symptom, and if it were as serious as was generally believed, there would be a great many more blind and insane people in the community than there were. The patient went away somewhat comforted, but at eleven o'clock—his first visit had been at nine—he was back again. He still saw the floating specks, and was still worried about them. I examined his eyes again as carefully as before, and again was able to assure him that there was nothing wrong with them. In the afternoon I was not in my office, but I was told that he was there at three and at five. At seven he came again, bringing with him his family physician, an old friend of mine. I said to the latter:

"Please make this patient stay at home. I have to charge him for his visits, because he is taking up so much of my time; but it is a shame to take his money when there is nothing wrong with him."

What my friend said to him I don't know, but he did not come back again.

I did not know as much about muscae volitantes then as I know now, or I might have saved both of these patients a great deal of uneasiness. I could tell them that

their eyes were normal, but I did not know how to relieve them of the symptom, which is simply an illusion
resulting from mental strain. The specks are associated
to a considerable extent with markedly imperfect eyesight, because persons whose eyesight is imperfect always strain to see; but persons whose eyesight is ordinarily normal may see them at times, because no eye has
normal sight all the time. Most people can see muscae
volitantes when they look at the sun, or any uniformly
bright surface, like a sheet of white paper upon which the
sun is shining. This is because most people strain when
they look at surfaces of this kind. The specks are never
seen, in short, except when the eyes and mind are under
a strain, and they always disappear when the strain is
relieved. If one can remember a small letter on the
Snellen test card by central fixation, the specks will immediately disappear, or cease to move; but if one tries
to remember two or more letters equally well at one
time, they will reappear and move.

Usually the strain that causes muscae volitantes is
very easily relieved. A school teacher who had been
annoyed by these appearances for years came to me because the condition had grown recently much worse. I
was able in half an hour to improve her sight, which had
been slightly myopic, to normal, whereupon the specks
disappeared. Next day they came back, but another
visit to the office brought relief. After that the patient
was able to carry out the treatment at home, and had
no more trouble.

A physician who suffered constantly from headaches
and muscae volitantes was able to read only 20/70 when
he looked at the Snellen test card, while the retinoscope
showed mixed astigmatism and he saw the specks.

When he looked at a blank wall, or a blank white card, the retinoscope still showed mixed astigmatism and he still saw the specks. When, however, he remembered a black spot as well as he could see it, when looking at these surfaces, there were no specks, and the retinoscope indicated no error of refraction. In a few days he obtained complete relief from the astigmatism, the muscae volitantes, and the headaches, as well as from chronic conjunctivitis. His eyes, which had been partly closed, opened wide, and the sclera became white and clear. He became able to read in moving trains with no inconvenience, and—what impressed him more than anything else—he also became able to sit up all night with patients without having any trouble with his eyes next day.

CHAPTER XXIV

HOME TREATMENT

IT is not always possible for patients to go to a competent physician for relief. As the method of treating eye defects presented in this book is new, it may be impossible to find a physician in the neighborhood who understands it; and the patient may not be able to afford the expense of a long journey, or to take the time for treatment away from home. To such persons I wish to say that it is possible for a large number of people to be cured of defective eyesight without the aid, either of a physician or of anyone else. They can cure themselves, and for this purpose it is not necessary that they should understand all that has been written in this book, or in any other book. All that is necessary is to follow a few simple directions.

Place a Snellen test card on the wall at a distance of ten, fourteen, or twenty feet, and devote half a minute a day, or longer, to reading the smallest letters you can see, with each eye separately, covering the other with the palm of the hand in such a way as to avoid touching the eyeball. Keep a record of the progress made, with the dates. The simplest way to do this is by the method used by oculists, who record the vision in the form of a fraction, with the distance at which the letter is read as the numerator and the distance at which it ought to be read as the denominator. The figures above, or to one side of, the lines of letters on the test card indicate the distance at which these letters should be read by persons with normal eyesight. Thus a vision of 10/200 would mean that the big C, which ought to be read at 200 feet, cannot be seen at a greater distance than ten feet. A vision of 20/10 would mean that the ten line, which the normal eye is not ordinarily expected to read at a greater distance than ten feet, is seen at double that distance. This is a standard commonly attained by persons who have practiced my methods.

Another and even better way to test the sight is to compare the blackness of the letter at the near-point and at the distance, in a dim light and in a good one. With perfect sight, black is not altered by illumination or distance. It appears just as black at the distance as at the near-point, and just as black in a dim light as in a good one. If it does not appear equally black to you under all these conditions, therefore, you may know that your sight is imperfect.

Children under twelve years who have not worn glasses are usually cured of defective eyesight by the above method in three months, six months, or a year. Adults who have never worn glasses are benefited in a very short time—a week or two—and if the trouble is not very bad, may be cured in the course of from three to six months. Children or adults who have worn glasses, however, are more difficult to relieve, and will usually have to practice the method of gaining relaxation described in other chapters; they will also have to devote considerable time to the treatment.

It is absolutely necessary that the glasses be discarded. No half-way measures can be tolerated, if a cure is desired. Do not attempt to wear weaker glasses, and do not wear glasses for emergencies. Persons who are unable to do without glasses for all purposes are not likely to be able to cure themselves.

Children and adults who have worn glasses will have to devote an hour or longer every day to practice with the test card and the balance of their time to practice on other objects. It will be well for such patients to have two test cards, one to be used at the near-point, where it can be seen best, and the other at ten or twenty feet. The patient will find it a great help to shift from the near card to the distant one, as the unconscious memory of the letters seen at the near-point helps to bring out those seen at the distance.

If you cannot obtain a test card, you can make one for yourself by painting black letters of appropriate size on a white card, or on a piece of white paper. The approximate diameter of these letters, reading from the top of the card to the bottom, is: 3½ in., 1¾ in., 1¼ in., ⅞ in., 1¹⁄₁₆ in., ½ in., ⅜ in., ¼ in., ³⁄₁₆ in.

If the patient can secure the aid of some person with normal sight, it will be a great advantage. In fact, persons whose cases are obstinate will find it very difficult, if not impossible, to cure themselves without the aid of a teacher. The teacher, if he is to benefit the patient, must himself be able to derive benefit from the various methods recommended. If his vision is 10/10, he must be able to improve it to 20/10, or more. If he can read fine print at twelve inches, he must become able to read it at six, or at three inches. He must also have sufficient control over his visual memory to relieve and prevent pain. A person who has defective sight, either for the distance or the near-point, and who cannot remember black well enough to relieve and prevent pain, will be unable to be of any material assistance in obstinate cases; and no one will be able to be of any assistance in the application of any method which he himself has not used successfully.

Parents who wish to preserve and improve the eye-sight of their children should encourage them to read the Snellen test card every day. There should, in fact, be a Snellen test card in every family; for when properly used it always prevents myopia and other errors of re-fraction, always improves the vision, even when this is already normal, and always benefits functional nervous troubles. Parents should improve their own eyesight to normal, so that their children may not imitate wrong methods of using the eyes and will not be subject to the influence of an atmosphere of strain. They should also learn the principles of central fixation sufficiently well to relieve and prevent pain, in order that they may teach their children to do the same. This practice not only makes it possible to avoid suffering, but is a great benefit to the general health.

CHAPTER XXV

CORRESPONDENCE TREATMENT

CORRESPONDENCE treatment is usually regarded as quackery, and it would be manifestly impossible to treat many diseases in this way. Pneumonia and typhoid, for instance, could not possibly be treated by correspondence, even if the physician had a sure cure for these conditions and the mails were not too slow for the purpose. In the case of most diseases, in fact, there are serious objections to correspondence treatment.

But myopia, hypermetropia and astigmatism are functional conditions, not organic, as the text-books teach and as I believed myself until I learned better. Their treatment by correspondence, therefore, has not the drawbacks that exist in the case of most physical derangements. One cannot, it is true, fit glasses by correspondence as well as when the patient is in the office, but even this can be done, as the following case illustrates.

An old colored woman in the wilds of Honduras, far removed from any physician or optician, was unable to read her Bible, and her son, a waiter in New York, asked me if I could not do something for her. The suggestion gave me a distinct shock which I will remember as long as I live. I had never dreamed of the possibility of prescribing glasses for anyone I had not seen, and I had, besides, some very disquieting recollections of colored women whom I had tried to fit with glasses at my clinic.

246

If I had so much difficulty in prescribing the proper glasses under favorable conditions, how could I be expected to fit a patient whom I could not even see? The waiter was deferentially persistent, however. He had more faith in my genius than I had, and as his mother was nearing the end of her life, he was very anxious to gratify her last wishes. So, like the unjust judge of the parable, I yielded at last to his importunity, and wrote a prescription for convex 3.00 D. S. The young man ordered the glasses and mailed them to his mother, and by return mail came a very grateful letter stating that they were perfectly satisfactory.

A little later the patient wrote that she couldn't see objects at the distance that were perfectly plain to other people, and asked if some glasses couldn't be sent that would make her see at the distance as well as she did at the near-point. This seemed a more difficult proposition than the first one; but again the son was persistent, and I myself could not get the old lady out of my mind. So again I decided to do what I could. The waiter had told me that his mother had read her Bible long after the age of forty. Therefore I knew she could not have much hypermetropia, and was probably slightly myopic. I knew also that she could not have much astigmatism, for in that case her sight would always have been noticeably imperfect. Accordingly I told her son to ask her to measure very accurately the distance between her eyes and the point at which she could read her Bible best with her glasses, and to send me the figures. In due time I received, not figures, but a piece of string about a quarter of an inch in diameter and exactly ten inches long. If the patient's vision had been normal for the distance, I knew that she would have been able to read her Bible best with her glasses at thirteen inches. The string showed that at ten inches she had a refraction of four diopters. Subtracting from this the three diopters of her reading glasses, I got one diopter of myopia. I accordingly wrote a prescription for concave 1.00 D. S., and the glasses were ordered and mailed to Honduras. The acknowledgment was even more grateful than in the case of the first pair. The patient said that for the first time in her life she was able to read signs and see other objects at a distance as well as other people did, and that the whole world looked entirely different to her.

Would anyone venture to say that it was unethical for me to try to help this patient? Would it have been better to leave her in her isolation without even the consolation of Bible reading? I do not think so. What I did for her required only an ordinary knowledge of physiological optics, and if I had failed, I could not have done her much harm.

In the case of the treatment of imperfect sight without glasses there can be even less objection to the correspondence method. It is true that in most cases progress is more rapid and the results more certain when the patient can be seen personally; but often this is impossible, and I see no reason why patients who cannot have the benefit of personal treatment should be denied such aid as can be given them by correspondence. I have been treating patients in this way for years, and often with extraordinary success.

Some years ago an English gentleman wrote to me that his glasses were very unsatisfactory. They not only did not give him good sight, but they increased, instead of lessening, his discomfort. He asked if I could help him, and since relaxation always relieves discomfort and improves the vision, I did not believe that I was doing him an injury in telling him how to rest his eyes. He followed my directions with such good results that in a short time he obtained perfect sight for both the distance and the near-point without glasses, and was completely relieved of his pain. Five years later he wrote me that he had qualified as a sharpshooter in the army. Did I do wrong in treating him by correspondence? I do not think so.

After the United States entered the European war, an officer wrote to me from the deserts of Arizona that the use of his eyes at the near-point caused him great discomfort, which glasses did not relieve, and that the strain had produced granulation of the lids. As it was impossible for him to come to New York, I undertook to treat him by correspondence. He improved very rapidly. The inflammation of the lids was relieved almost immediately, and in about four months he wrote me that he had read one of my own reprints—by no means a short one—in a dim light, with no bad after effects; that the glare of the Arizona sun, with the Government thermometer registering 114, did not annoy him; and that he could read the ten line on the test card at fifteen feet almost perfectly, while even at twenty feet he was able to make out most of the letters.

A third case was that of a forester in the employ of the U. S. Government. He had myopic astigmatism, and suffered extreme discomfort, which was not relieved either by glasses or by long summers in the mountains, where he used his eyes but little for close work. He was unable to come to New York for treatment, and although I told him that correspondence treatment was somewhat uncertain, he said he was willing to risk it. It took three days for his letters to reach me and another three for my reply to reach him, and as letters were not always written promptly on either side, he often did not hear from me more than once in three weeks. Progress under these conditions was necessarily slow; but his discomfort was relieved very quickly, and in about ten months his sight had improved from 20/50 to 20/20.

In almost every case the treatment of patients coming from a distance is continued by correspondence after they return to their homes; and although they do not get on so well as when they are coming to the office, they usually continue to make progress until they are cured.

At the same time it is often very difficult to make patients understand what they should do when one has to communicate with them entirely by writing, and probably all would get on better if they could have some personal treatment. At the present time the number of doctors in different parts of the United States who understand the treatment of imperfect sight without glasses is altogether too few, and my efforts to interest them in the matter have not been very successful.

CHAPTER XXVI

THE PREVENTION OF MYOPIA IN SCHOOLS: METHODS THAT FAILED

N O phase of ophthalmology, not even the problem of accommodation, has been the subject of so much investigation and discussion as the cause and prevention of myopia. Since hypermetropia was supposed to be due to a congenital deformation of the eyeball, and astigmatism, until recently, was also supposed to be congenital in most cases, these conditions were not thought to call for any explanation, nor to admit of any prevention; but myopia appeared to be acquired. It therefore presented a problem of immense practical importance to which many eminent men devoted years of labor.

Voluminous statistics were collected regarding its occurrence, and are still being collected. The subject has produced libraries of literature. But very little light is to be gained from the perusal of this material, and for the most part it leaves the reader with an impression of hopeless confusion. It is impossible even to arrive at any conclusion as to the prevalence of the complaint; for not only has there been no uniformity of standards and methods, but none of the investigators has taken into account the fact that the refraction of the eye is not a constant condition, but one which continually varies. There is no doubt, however, that most children, when they begin school, are free from this defect, and that both the number of cases and the degree of the myopia steadily increase as the educational process progresses. Professor Hermann Cohn, of Breslau, whose report of his study of the eyes of upwards of 10,000 children first called general attention to this subject, found scarcely one per cent of myopia in the village schools, twenty to forty per cent in the "Realschulen," thirty to thirty-five in the gymnasia, and fifty-three to sixty-four in the professional schools. His investigations were repeated in many cities of Europe and America, and his observations, with some difference in percentages, everywhere confirmed.

These conditions were unanimously attributed to the excessive use of the eyes for near work, though, according to the theory that the lens is the agent of accommodation, it was a little difficult to see just why near work should have this effect. On the supposition that accommodation was effected by an elongation of the eyeball, it would have been easy to understand why an excessive amount of accommodation should produce a permanent elongation. But why should an abnormal demand on the accommodative power of the lens produce a change, not in the shape of that body, but in that of the eyeball? Numerous answers to this question have been proposed, but no one has yet succeeded in finding a satisfactory one.[1] In the case of children it has been assumed by many authorities that, since the coats of the eye are softer in youth than in later years, they are unable to withstand a supposed intraocular tension produced by near work. When other errors of refraction, such as hypermetropia and astigmatism, believed to be congenital, were present, it has been supposed that the accommodative struggle for distinct vision produced irritation and strain which encouraged the production of short-

---

[1] A satisfactory explanation of the mechanism by which near work produces myopia has not yet been given.—Tscherning: Physiologic Optics, p. 86.

It is not yet determined how near work changes the longitudinal structure of the eye.—Eversbusch: The Diseases of Children, vol. vi, p. 291.

sight. When the condition developed in adults, the explanations had to be modified to fit the case, and the fact that a considerable number of cases were observed among peasants and others who did not use their eyes for near work led some authorities to divide the anomaly into two classes, one caused by near work and one unrelated to it, the latter being conveniently attributed to hereditary tendencies.

As it was impossible to abandon the educational system, attempts were made to minimize the supposed evil effects of the reading, writing and other near work which it demanded. Careful and detailed rules were laid down by various authorities as to the sizes of type to be used in schoolbooks, the length of the lines, their distance apart, the distance at which the book should be held, the amount and arrangement of the light, the construction of the desks, the length of time the eyes might be used without a change of focus, etc. Face-rests were even devised to hold the eyes at the prescribed distance from the desk and to prevent stooping, which was supposed to cause congestion of the eyeball and thus to encourage elongation. The Germans, with characteristic thoroughness, actually used these instruments of torture, Cohn never allowing his own children to write without one, "even when sitting at the best possible desk."[1]

The results of these preventive measures were disappointing. Some observers reported a slight decrease in the percentage of myopia in schools in which the prescribed reforms had been made, but on the whole, as Risley has observed in his discussion of the subject in Norris and Oliver's "System of Diseases of the Eye," "the injurious results of the educational process were not notably arrested."

---

[1] The Hygiene of the Eye in Schools, p. 127.

"It is a significant, though discouraging, fact," he continues, "that the increase, as found by Cohn, both in the percentage and in the degree of myopia, had taken place in those schools where he had especially exerted himself to secure the introduction of hygienic reforms; and the

Fig. 56.   Face-Rest Designed by Kallmann, a German
Optician

Cohn never allowed his children to write without it, even when sitting at the best possible desk.

same is true of the observations of Just, who had examined the eyes of twelve hundred and twenty-nine of the pupils of the two high schools of Zittau, in both of which the hygienic conditions were all that could be desired. He found, nevertheless, that the excellent arrangements had not in any degree lessened the percentage of increase in myopia."[1]

---

[1] School Hygiene, System of Diseases of the Eye, vol. ii, p. 361.

Further study of the subject has only added to its difficulty, while at the same time it has tended to relieve the schools of much of the responsibility formerly attributed to them for the production of myopia. As the "American Encyclopedia of Ophthalmology" points out, "the theory that myopia is due to close work aggravated by town life and badly lighted rooms is gradually giving ground before statistics."[1]

In an investigation in London, for instance, in which the schools were carefully selected to reveal any differences that might arise from the various influences, hygienic, social and racial, to which the children were subjected, the proportion of myopia in the best lighted building of the group was actually found to be higher than in the one where the lighting conditions were worst. although the higher degrees of myopia were more numerous in the latter than in the former. It has also been found that there is just as much myopia in schools where little near work is done as in those in which the demand upon the accommodative power of the eye is greater.[2] It is only a minority of children, moreover, that become myopic; yet all are subject to practically the same influences, and even in the same child one eye may become myopic while the other remains normal. On the theory that shortsight results from any external influence to which the eye is exposed, it is impossible to account for the fact that under the same conditions of life the eyes of different individuals and the two eyes of the same individual behave differently.

Owing to the difficulty of reconciling these facts on the basis of the earlier theories, there is now a growing

[1] American Encyclopedia and Dictionary of Ophthalmology, edited by Wood, 1913-1919, vol. xi, p. 8271.
[2] Lawson: Brit. Med. Jour., June 18, 1898.

disposition to attribute myopia to hereditary tendencies;[1] but no satisfactory evidence on this point has been brought forward, and the fact that primitive peoples who have always had good eyesight become myopic just as quickly as any others when subjected to the conditions of civilized life, like the Indian pupils at Carlisle,[2] seems to be conclusive evidence against it.

In spite of the repeated failure of preventive measures based upon the limitation of near work and the regulation of lighting, desks, types, etc., the use of the eyes at the near-point under unfavorable conditions is still admitted by most exponents of the heredity theory as probably, if not certainly, a secondary cause of myopia. Sidler-Huguenin, however, whose startling conclusions as to the hopelessness of controlling shortsight were quoted earlier, has observed so little benefit from such precautions that he believes a myope may become an engineer just as well as a farmer, or a forester; and as a result of his experiences with anisometropes, persons with an inequality of refraction between the two organs of vision, he even suggests that the use of myopic eyes may possibly be more favorable to their well-being than their non-use. In 150 cases in which, owing to this inequality and other conditions, the subjects practically used but one eye, the weaker organ, he reports, became gradually more and more myopic, sometimes excessively so, in open defiance of all the accepted theories relating to the matter.

The prevalence of myopia, the unsatisfactoriness of

---

[1] It seems to have been amply demonstrated, by the studies of Motais, Steiger, Miss Barrington, and Karl Pearson, that errors of refraction are inherited. And while the use of the eyes for near work is probably a secondary cause, determining largely the development of the defect, it is not the primary cause.—Cyclopedia of Education, edited by Monroe, 1911-1913, vol. iv, p. 361.

[2] Fox (quoted by Risley): System of Diseases of the Eye, vol. ii, p. 357.

all explanations of its origin, and the futility of all methods of prevention, have led some writers of repute to the conclusion that the elongated eyeball is a natural physiological adaptation to the needs of civilization. Against this view two unanswerable arguments can be brought. One is that the myopic eye does not see so well even at the near-point as the normal eye, and the other that the defect tends to progression with very serious results, often ending in blindness. If Nature has attempted to adapt the eye to civilized conditions by an elongation of the globe, she has done it in a very clumsy manner. It is true that many authorities assume the existence of two kinds of myopia, one physiological, or at least harmless, and the other pathological; but since it is impossible to say with certainty whether a given case is going to progress or not, this distinction, even if it were correct, would be more important theoretically than practically.

Into such a slough of despair and contradiction have the misdirected labors of a hundred years led us! But in the light of truth the problem turns out to be a very simple one. In view of the facts given in Chapters V and IX, it is easy to understand why all previous attempts to prevent myopia have failed. All these attempts have aimed at lessening the strain of near work upon the eye, leaving the strain to see distant objects unaffected, and totally ignoring the mental strain which underlies the optical one. There are many differences between the conditions to which the children of primitive man were subjected, and those under which the offspring of civilized races spend their developing years, besides the mere fact that the latter learn things out of books and write things on paper, and the former did not. In the process of education, civilized children are shut up for hours every day within four walls, in the charge of teachers who are too often nervous and irritable. They are even compelled to remain for long periods in the same position. The things they are required to learn may be presented in such a way as to be excessively uninteresting; and they are under a continual compulsion to think of the gaining of marks and prizes rather than the acquisition of knowledge for its own sake. Some children endure these unnatural conditions better than others. Many cannot stand the strain, and thus the schools become the hotbed, not only of myopia, but of all other errors of refraction.

CHAPTER XXVII

THE PREVENTION AND CURE OF MYOPIA AND OTHER ERRORS OF REFRACTION IN SCHOOLS: A METHOD THAT SUCCEEDED

YOU cannot see anything with perfect sight unless you have seen it before. When the eye looks at an unfamiliar object it always strains more or less to see that object, and an error of refraction is always produced. When children look at unfamiliar writing or figures on the blackboard, distant maps, diagrams, or pictures, the retinoscope always shows that they are myopic, though their vision may be under other circumstances absolutely normal. The same thing happens when adults look at unfamiliar distant objects. When the eye regards a familiar object, however, the effect is quite otherwise. Not only can it be regarded without strain, but the strain of looking later at unfamiliar objects is lessened.

This fact furnishes us with a means of overcoming the mental strain to which children are subjected by the modern educational system. It is impossible to see anything perfectly when the mind is under a strain, and if children become able to relax when looking at familiar objects, they become able, sometimes in an incredibly brief space of time, to maintain their relaxation when looking at unfamiliar objects.

I discovered this fact while examining the eyes of 1,500 school children at Grand Forks, N. D., in 1903.[1] In

---

[1] Bates: The Prevention of Myopia in School Children, N. Y. Med. Jour., July 29, 1911.

many cases, children who could not read all of the letters on the Snellen test card at the first test read them at the second or third test. After a class had been examined, the children who had failed would sometimes ask for a second test, and then it often happened that they would read the whole card with perfect vision. So frequent were these occurrences that there was no escaping the conclusion that in some way the vision was improved by reading the Snellen test card. In one class I found a boy who at first appeared to be very myopic, but who, after a little encouragement, read all the letters on the test card. The teacher asked me about this boy's vision, because she had found him to be very "nearsighted." When I said that his vision was normal she was incredulous, and suggested that he might have learned the letters by heart, or been prompted by another pupil. He was unable to read the writing or figures on the blackboard, she said, or to see the maps, charts and diagrams on the walls, and did not recognize people across the street. She asked me to test his sight again, which I did, very carefully, under her supervision, the sources of error which she had suggested being eliminated. Again the boy read all the letters on the card. Then the teacher tested his sight. She wrote some words and figures on the blackboard, and asked him to read them. He did so correctly. Then she wrote additional words and figures, which he read equally well. Finally she asked him to tell the hour by the clock, twenty-five feet distant, which he did correctly. It was a dramatic situation, both the teacher and the children being intensely interested. Three other cases in the class were similar, their vision, which had previously been very defective for distant objects, becoming normal in the few moments devoted to testing their eyes. It is not surprising that after such a demonstration the teacher asked to have a Snellen test card placed permanently in the room. The children were directed to read the smallest letters they could see from their seats at least once every day, with both eyes together and with each eye separately, the other being covered with the palm of the hand in such a way as to avoid pressure on the eyeball. Those whose vision was defective were encouraged to read it more frequently, and, in fact, needed no encouragement to do so after they found that the practice helped them to see the blackboard, and stopped the headaches, or other discomfort, previously resulting from the use of their eyes.

In another class of forty children, between six and eight, thirty of the pupils gained normal vision while their eyes were being tested. The remainder were cured later under the supervision of the teacher by exercises in distant vision with the Snellen card. This teacher had noted every year for fifteen years that at the opening of the school in the fall all the children could see the writing on the blackboard from their seats, but before school closed the following spring all of them without exception complained that they could not see it at a distance of more than ten feet. After learning of the benefits to be derived from the daily practice of distant vision with familiar objects as the points of fixation, this teacher kept a Snellen test card continually in her classroom and directed the children to read it every day. The result was that for eight years no more of the children under her care acquired defective eyesight.

This teacher had attributed the invariable deterioration in the eyesight of her charges during the school year to the fact that her classroom was in the basement and the

light poor.   But teachers with well-lighted classrooms
had the same experience, and after the Snellen test card
was introduced into both the well-lighted and the poorly
lighted rooms, and the children read it every day, the deterioration of their eyesight not only ceased, but the vision of all improved.   Vision which had been below
normal improved, in most cases, to normal, while children
who already had normal sight, usually reckoned at 20/20,
became able to read 20/15, or 20/10.   And not only was
myopia cured, but the vision for near objects was improved.

At the request of the superintendent of the schools of
Grand Forks, Mr. J. Nelson Kelly, the system was introduced into all the schools of the city and was used continuously for eight years, during which time it reduced
myopia among the children, which I found at the beginning to be about six per cent, to less than one per cent.

In 1911 and 1912 the same system was introduced into
some of the schools of New York City,[1] with an attend-
ance of about ten thousand children.   Many of the teachers neglected to use the cards, being unable to believe
that such a simple method, and one so entirely at vari-
ance with previous teaching on the subject, could accomplish the desired results.   Others kept the cards in a
closet except when they were needed for the daily eye
drill, lest the children should memorize them.   Thus they
not only put an unnecessary burden upon themselves, but
did what they could to defeat the purpose of the system,
which is to give the children daily exercise in distant vision with a familiar object as the point of fixation.   A
considerable number, however, used the system intel-
ligently and persistently, and in less than a year were

---

[1] Bates: Myopia Prevention by Teachers, N. Y. Med. Jour., Aug. 30, 1913.

able to present reports showing that of three thousand children with imperfect sight, over one thousand had obtained normal vision by its means. Some of these children, as in the case of the children of Grand Forks, were cured in a few minutes. Many of the teachers were also cured, some of them very quickly. In some cases the results of the system were so astonishing as to be scarcely credible.

In a class of mental defectives, where the teacher had kept records of the eyesight of the children for several years, it had been invariably found that their vision grew steadily worse as the term advanced. As soon as the Snellen test card had been introduced, however, they began to improve. Then came a doctor from the Board of Health who tested the eyes of the children and put glasses on all of them, even those whose sight was fairly good. The use of the card was then discontinued, as the teacher did not consider it proper to interfere while the children were wearing glasses prescribed by a physician. Very soon, however, the children began to lose, break, or discard their glasses. Some said that the spectacles gave them headaches, or that they felt better without them. In the course of a month or so most of the aids to vision which the Board of Health had supplied had disappeared. The teacher then felt herself at liberty to resume the use of the Snellen test card. Its benefits were immediate. The eyesight and the mentality of the children improved simultaneously, and soon they were all drafted into the regular classes, because it was found that they were making the same progress in their studies as the other children were.

Another teacher reported an equally interesting experience. She had a class of children who did not fit into the other grades. Many of them were backward in their studies. Some were persistent truants. All of them had defective eyesight. A Snellen test card was hung in the classroom where all the children could see it, and the teacher carried out my instructions literally. At the end of six months all but two had been cured, and these had improved very much, while the worst incorrigible and the worst truant had become good students. The incorrigible, who had previously refused to study, because, he said, it gave him a headache to look at a book, or at the blackboard, found out that the test card, in some way, did him a lot of good; and although the teacher had asked him to read it but once a day, he read it whenever he felt uncomfortable. The result was that in a few weeks his vision had become normal and his objection to study had disappeared. The truant had been in the habit of remaining away from school two or three days every week, and neither his parents nor the truant officer had been able to do anything about it. To the great surprise of his teacher he never missed a day after having begun to read the Snellen test card. When she asked for an explanation, he told her that what had driven him away from school was the pain that came in his eyes whenever he tried to study, or to read the writing on the blackboard. After reading the Snellen test card, he said, his eyes and head were rested and he was able to read without any discomfort.

To remove any doubts that might arise as to the cause of the improvement noted in the eyesight of the children, comparative tests were made with and without cards. In one case six pupils with defective sight were examined daily for one week without the use of the test card. No improvement took place. The card was then restored to its place, and the group was instructed to read it every day. At the end of a week all had improved and five were cured. In the case of another group of defectives the results were similar. During the week that the card was not used, no improvement was noted; but after a week of exercises in distant vision with the card all showed marked improvement, and at the end of a month all were cured. In order that there might be no question as to the reliability of the records of the teachers, some of the principals asked the Board of Health to send an inspector to test the vision of the pupils, and whenever this was done the records were found to be correct.

One day I visited the city of Rochester, and while there I called on the Superintendent of Public Schools and told him about my method of preventing myopia. He was very much interested and invited me to introduce it in one of his schools. I did so, and at the end of three months a report was sent to me showing that the vision of all the children had improved, while quite a number of them had obtained normal vision in both eyes.

The method has been used in a number of other cities and always with the same result. The vision of all the children improved, and many of them obtained normal vision in the course of a few minutes, days, weeks, or months.

It is difficult to prove a negative proposition, but since this system improved the vision of all the children who used it, it follows that none could have grown worse. It is therefore obvious that it must have prevented myopia. This cannot be said of any method of preventing myopia in schools which had previously been tried. All other methods are based on the idea that it is the excessive use of the eyes for near work that causes myopia, and all of them have admittedly failed.

It is also obvious that the method must have prevented

other errors of refraction, a problem which previously had not even been seriously considered, because hypermetropia is supposed to be congenital, and astigmatism was until recently supposed also to be congenital in the great majority of cases. Anyone who knows how to use a retinoscope may, however, demonstrate in a few minutes that both of these conditions are acquired; for no matter how astigmatic or hypermetropic an eye may be, its vision always becomes normal when it looks at a blank surface without trying to see. It may also be demonstrated that when children are learning to read, write, draw, sew, or to do anything else that necessitates their looking at unfamiliar objects at the near-point, hypermetropia, or hypermetropic astigmatism, is always produced. The same is true of adults. These facts have not been reported before, so far as I am aware, and they strongly suggest that children need, first of all, eye education. They must be able to look at strange letters or objects at the near-point without strain before they can make much progress in their studies, and in every case in which the method has been tried it has been proven that this end is attained by daily exercise in distant vision with the Snellen test card. When their distant vision has been improved by this means, children invariably become able to use their eyes without strain at the near-point.

The method succeeded best when the teacher did not wear glasses. In fact, the effect upon the children of a teacher who wears glasses is so detrimental that no such person should be allowed to be a teacher, and since errors of refraction are curable, such a ruling would work no hardship on anyone. Not only do children imitate the visual habits of a teacher who wears glasses, but the nervous strain of which the defective sight is an expression produces in them a similar condition. In classes of the same grade, with the same lighting, the sight of children whose teachers did not wear glasses has always been found to be better than the sight of children whose teachers did wear them. In one case I tested the sight of children whose teacher wore glasses, and found it very imperfect. The teacher went out of the room on an errand, and after she had gone I tested them again. The results were very much better. When the teacher returned she asked about the sight of a particular boy, a very nervous child, and as I was proceeding to test him she stood before him and said, "Now, when the doctor tells you to read the card, do it." The boy couldn't see anything. Then she went behind him, and the effect was the same as if she had left the room. The boy read the whole card.

Still better results would be obtained if we could reorganize the educational system on a rational basis. Then we might expect a general return of that primitive acuity of vision which we marvel at so greatly when we read about it in the memoirs of travellers. But even under existing conditions it has proven beyond the shadow of a doubt that errors of refraction are no necessary part of the price we must pay for education.

There are at least ten million children in the schools of the United States who have defective sight. This condition prevents them from taking full advantage of the educational opportunities which the State provides. It undermines their health and wastes the taxpayers' money. If allowed to continue, it will be an expense and a handicap to them throughout their lives. In many cases it will be a source of continual misery and suffering. And yet practically all of these cases could be cured and the development of new ones prevented by the daily reading of the Snellen test card.

Why should our children be compelled to suffer and wear glasses for want of this simple measure of relief? It costs practically nothing. In fact, it would not be necessary, in some cases, as in the schools of New York City, even to purchase the Snellen test cards, as they are already being used to test the eyes of the children. Not only does it place practically no additional burden upon the teachers, but, by improving the eyesight, health, disposition and mentality of their pupils, it greatly lightens their labors. No one would venture to suggest, further, that it could possibly do any harm. Why, then, should there be any delay about introducing it into the schools? If there is still thought to be need for further investigation and discussion, we can investigate and discuss just as well after the children get the cards as before, and by adopting that course we shall not run the risk of needlessly condemning another generation to that curse which heretofore has always dogged the footsteps of civilization, namely, defective eyesight. I appeal to all who read these lines to use whatever influence they possess toward the attainment of this end.

DIRECTIONS

FOR USING THE SNELLEN TEST CARD FOR THE PREVENTION AND CURE OF IMPERFECT SIGHT IN SCHOOLS

The Snellen Test Card is placed permanently upon the wall of the classroom, and every day the children silently read the smallest letters they can see from their seats with each eye separately, the other being covered with the palm of the hand in such a way as to avoid pressure on the eyeball. This takes no appreciable amount of time and is sufficient to improve the sight of all children in one week and to cure all errors of refraction after some months, a year, or longer.

Children with markedly defective vision should be encouraged to read the card more frequently. Children wearing glasses should not be interfered with, as they are supposed to be under the care of a physician, and the practice will do them little or no good while the glasses are worn.

While not essential, it is a great advantage to have records made of the vision of each pupil at the time when the method is introduced, and thereafter at convenient intervals—annually or more frequently. This may be done by the teacher.

The records should include the name and age of the pupils, the vision of each eye tested at twenty feet, and the date. For example:

> John Smith, 10, Sept. 15, 1919
> R. V. (vision of the right eye) 20/40
> L. V. (vision of the left eye) 20/20
>
> John Smith, 11, January 1, 1920
> R. V. 20/30
> L. V. 20/15

A certain amount of supervision is absolutely necessary. At least once a year some one who understands the method should visit each classroom for the purpose of answering questions, encouraging the teachers to continue the use of the method, and making some kind of a report to the proper authorities. It is not necessary that either the supervisor, the teachers, or the children should understand anything about the physiology of the eye.

CHAPTER XXVIII

THE STORY OF EMILY

THE efficacy of the method of treating imperfect sight without glasses presented in this book has been demonstrated in thousand of cases, not only in my own practice but in that of many persons of whom I may not even have heard; for almost all patients, when they are cured, proceed to cure others. At a social gathering one evening a lady told me that she had met a number of my patients; but when she mentioned their names I found that I did not remember any of them and said so.

"That is because you cured them by proxy," she said. "You didn't directly cure Mrs. Jones or Mrs. Brown, but you cured Mrs. Smith, and Mrs. Smith cured the other ladies. You didn't treat Mr. and Mrs. Simpkins, or Mr. Simpkins' mother and brother, but you may remember that you cured Mr. Simpkins' boy of a squint, and he cured the rest of the family."

In schools where the Snellen test card was used to prevent and cure imperfect sight, the children, after they were cured themselves, often took to the practice of ophthalmology with the greatest enthusiasm and success, curing their fellow students, their parents and their friends. They made a kind of game of the treatment, and the progress of each school case was watched with the most intense interest by all the children. On a bright day, when the patients saw well, there was great rejoicing, and on a dark day there was corresponding depression. One girl cured twenty-six children in six months; another cured twelve in three months; a third developed quite a varied ophthalmological practice, and did things of which older and more experienced practitioners might well have been proud. Going to the school which she attended one day, I asked this girl about her sight, which had been very imperfect. She replied that it was now very good and that her headaches were quite gone. I tested her sight and found it normal. Then another child whose sight had also been very poor spoke up.

"I can see all right, too," she said. "Emily"—indicating girl No. 1—"cured me."

"Indeed!" I replied. "How did she do that?"

The second girl explained that Emily had had her read the card, which she could not see at all from the back of the room, at a distance of a few feet. The next day she had moved it a little farther away, and so on, until the patient was able to read it from the back of the room, just as the other children did. Emily now told her to cover the right eye and read the card with her left, and both girls were considerably upset to find that the uncovered eye was apparently blind. The school doctor was consulted and said that nothing could be done. The eye had been blind from birth and no treatment would do any good.

Nothing daunted, however, Emily undertook the treatment. She told the patient to cover her good eye and go up close to the card, and at a distance of a foot or less it was found that she could read even the small letters. The little practitioner then proceeded confidently as with the other eye, and after many months of practice the patient became the happy possessor of normal vision in both eyes. The case had, in fact, been simply one of high myopia, and the school doctor, not being a specialist, had not detected the difference between this condition and blindness.

In the same classroom there had been a little girl with congenital cataract, but on the occasion of my visit the defect had disappeared.   This, too, it appeared, was Emily's doing.   The school doctor had said that there was no help for this eye except through operation, and as the sight of the other eye was pretty good, he fortunately did not think it necessary to urge such a course. Emily accordingly took the matter in hand.   She had the patient stand close to the card, where, with the good eye covered, she was unable to see even the big C.   Emily now held the card between the patient and the light, and moved it back and forth.   At a distance of three or four feet this movement could be observed indistinctly by the patient.   The card was then moved farther away, until the patient became able to see it move at ten feet and to see some of the larger letters indistinctly at a less distance.   Finally, after six months, she became able to read the card with the bad eye as well as with the good one. After testing her sight and finding it normal in both eyes, I said to Emily:

"You are a splendid doctor.   You beat them all.   Have you done anything else?"

The child blushed, and turning to another of her classmates, said:

"Mamie, come here."

Mamie stepped forward and I looked at her eyes. There appeared to be nothing wrong with them.

"I cured her," said Emily.

"What of?" I inquired.

"Cross eyes," replied Emily.

"How?" I asked, with growing astonishment.

Emily described a procedure very similar to that adopted in the other cases.   Finding that the sight of the crossed eye was very poor, so much so, indeed, that poor

Mamie could see practically nothing with it, the obvious course of action seemed to her to be the restoration of its sight; and, never having read any medical literature, she did not know that this was impossible. So she went to it. She had Mamie cover her good eye and practice the bad one at home and at school, until at last the sight became normal and the eye straight. The school doctor had wanted to have the eye operated upon, I was told, but, fortunately, Mamie was "scared" and would not consent. And here she was with two perfectly good, straight eyes.

"Anything else?" I inquired, when Mamie's case had been disposed of. Emily blushed again, and said:

"Here's Rose. Her eyes used to hurt her all the time, and she couldn't see anything on the blackboard. Her headaches used to be so bad that she had to stay away from school every once in a while. The doctor gave her glasses, but they didn't help her and she wouldn't wear them. When you told us the card would help our eyes I got busy with her. I had her read the card close up, and then I moved it farther away, and now she can see all right and her head doesn't ache any more. She comes to school every day, and we all thank you very much."

This was a case of compound hypermetropic astigmatism.

Such stories might be multiplied indefinitely. Emily's astonishing record might not possibly be duplicated, but lesser cures by cured patients have been very numerous, and serve to show that the benefits of the method of preventing and curing defects of vision in the schools which is presented in the foregoing chapter would be far-reaching. Not only errors of refraction would be cured, but many more serious defects; and not only the children would be helped, but their families and friends also.

CHAPTER XXIX

MIND AND VISION

POOR sight is admitted to be one of the most fruitful causes of retardation in the schools. It is estimated[1] that it may reasonably be held responsible for a quarter of the habitually "left-backs," and it is commonly assumed that all this might be prevented by suitable glasses.

There is much more involved in defective vision, however, than mere inability to see the blackboard or to use the eyes without pain or discomfort. Defective vision is the result of an abnormal condition of the mind, and when the mind is in an abnormal condition it is obvious that none of the processes of education can be conducted with advantage. By putting glasses upon a child we may, in some cases, neutralize the effect of this condition upon the eyes, and by making the patient more comfortable may improve his mental faculties to some extent; but we do not alter fundamentally the condition of the mind, and by confirming it in a bad habit we may make it worse.

It can easily be demonstrated that among the faculties of the mind which are impaired when the vision is impaired is the memory; and as a large part of the educational process consists of storing the mind with facts, and all the other mental processes depend upon one's

---

[1] School Health News, published by the Department of Health of New York City, February, 1919.

knowledge of facts, it is easy to see how little is accomplished by merely putting glasses on a child that has "trouble with its eyes." The extraordinary memory of primitive people has been attributed to the fact that owing to the absence of any convenient means of making written records they had to depend upon their memories, which were strengthened accordingly; but in view of the known facts about the relation of memory to eyesight it is more reasonable to suppose that the retentive memory of primitive man was due to the same cause as his keen vision, namely, a mind at rest.

The primitive memory, as well as primitive keenness of vision, has been found among civilized people; and if the necessary tests had been made it would doubtless have been found that they always occur together, as they did in a case which recently came under my observation. The subject was a child of ten with such marvelous eyesight that she could see the moons of Jupiter with the naked eye a fact which was demonstrated by her drawing a diagram of these satellites which exactly corresponded to the diagrams made by persons who had used a telescope. Her memory was equally remarkable. She could recite the whole content of a book after reading it, as Lord Macaulay is said to have done, and she learned more Latin in a few days without a teacher than her sister, who had six diopters of myopia, had been able to do in several years. She remembered five years afterward what she ate at a restaurant, she called the name of the waiter, the number of the building and the street in which it stood. She also remembered what she wore on this occasion and what every one else in the party wore. The same was true of every other event which had awakened her interest in any way, and it was a favorite amusement in her family to ask her what the menu had been and what people had worn on particular occasions.

When the sight of two persons is different it has been found that their memories differ in exactly the same degree. Two sisters, one of whom had only ordinary good vision, indicated by the formula 20/20, while the other had 20/10, found that the time it took them to learn eight verses of a poem varied in almost exactly the same ratio as their sight. The one whose vision was 20/10 learned eight verses of the poem in fifteen minutes, while the one whose vision was only 20/20 required thirty-one minutes to do the same thing. After palming, the one with ordinary vision learned eight more verses in twenty-one minutes, while the one with 20/10 was able to reduce her time by only two minutes, a variation clearly within the limits of error. In other words, the mind of the latter being already in a normal or nearly normal condition, she could not improve it appreciably by palming, while the former, whose mind was under a strain, was able to gain relaxation, and hence improve her memory, by this means.

Even when the difference in sight is between the two eyes of the same person, it can be demonstrated, as was pointed out in the chapter on "Memory as an Aid to Vision," that there is a corresponding difference in the memory, according to whether both eyes are open, or the better eye closed.

Under the present educational system there is a constant effort to compel the children to remember. These efforts always fail. They spoil both the memory and the sight. The memory cannot be forced any more than the vision can be forced. We remember without effort, just as we see without effort, and the harder we try to remember or see the less we are able to do so.

The sort of things we remember are the things that interest us, and the reason children have difficulty in learning their lessons is because they are bored by them. For the same reason, among others, their eyesight becomes impaired, boredom being a condition of mental strain in which it is impossible for the eye to function normally.

Some of the various kinds of compulsion now employed in the educational process may have the effect of awakening interest. Betty Smith's interest in winning a prize, for instance, or in merely getting ahead of Johnny Jones, may have the effect of rousing her interest in lessons that have hitherto bored her, and this interest may develop into a genuine interest in the acquisition of knowledge; but this cannot be said of the various fear incentives still so largely employed by teachers. These, on the contrary, have the effect, usually, of completely paralyzing minds already benumbed by lack of interest, and the effect upon the vision is equally disastrous.

The fundamental reason, both for poor memory and poor eyesight in school children, in short, is our irrational and unnatural educational system. Montessori has taught us that it is only when children are interested that they can learn. It is equally true that it is only when they are interested that they can see. This fact was strikingly illustrated in the case of one of the two pairs of sisters mentioned above. Phebe, of the keen eyes, who could recite whole books if she happened to be interested in them, disliked mathematics and anatomy extremely, and not only could not learn them but became myopic when they were presented to her mind. She could read letters a quarter of an inch high at twenty feet in a poor light, but when asked to read figures one to two inches high in a good light at ten feet she miscalled half of them. When asked to tell how much 2 and 3 made she said "4," before finally deciding on "5;" and all the time she was occupied with this disagreeable subject the retinoscope showed that she was myopic. When I asked her to look into my eye with the ophthalmoscope, she could see nothing, although a much lower degree of visual acuity is required to note the details of the interior of the eye than to see the moons of Jupiter.

Shortsighted Isabel, on the contrary, had a passion for mathematics and anatomy and excelled in those subjects. She learned to use the ophthalmoscope as easily as Phebe had learned Latin. Almost immediately she saw the optic nerve, and noted that the center was whiter than the periphery. She saw the light-colored lines, the arteries; and the darker ones, the veins; and she saw the light streaks on the blood-vessels. Some specialists never become able to do this, and no one could do it without normal vision. Isabel's vision, therefore, must have been temporarily normal when she did it. Her vision for figures, although not normal, was better than for letters.

In both these cases the ability to learn and the ability to see went hand in hand with interest. Phebe could read a photographic reduction of the Bible and recite what she had read verbatum, she could see the moons of Jupiter and draw a diagram of them afterwards, because she was interested in these things; but she could not see the interior of the eye, nor see figures even half as well as she saw letters, because these things bored her. When, however, it was suggested to her that it would be a good joke to surprise her teachers, who were always reproaching her for her backwardness in mathematics, by taking a high mark in a coming examination, her interest in the subject awakened and she contrived to learn enough to get seventy-eight per cent. In Isabel's case letters were antagonistic. She was not interested in most of the subjects with which they dealt, and therefore she was backward in those subjects and had become habitually myopic. But when asked to look at objects which aroused an intense interest her vision became normal.

When one is not interested, in short, one's mind is not under control, and without mental control one can neither learn nor see. Not only the memory but all other mental faculties are improved when the eyesight becomes normal. It is a common experience with patients cured of defective sight to find that their ability to do their work has improved.

The teacher whose letter is quoted in a later chapter testified that after gaining perfect eyesight she "knew better how to get at the minds of the pupils," was "more direct, more definite, less diffused, less vague," possessed, in fact, "central fixation of the mind." In another letter she said: "The better my eyesight becomes, the greater is my ambition. On the days when my sight is best I have the greatest anxiety to do things."

Another teacher reported that one of her pupils used to sit doing nothing all day long and apparently was not interested in anything. After the test card was introduced into the classroom and his sight improved, he became anxious to learn, and speedily developed into one of the best students in the class. In other words, his eyes and his mind became normal together.

A bookkeeper nearly seventy years of age who had

worn glasses for forty years found after he had gained
perfect sight without glasses that he could work more
rapidly and accurately and with less fatigue than ever
in his life before. During busy seasons, or when short
of help, he has worked for some weeks at a time from
7 a. m. until 11 p. m., and he insisted that he felt less
tired at night after he was through than he did in the
morning when he started. Previously, although he had
done more work than any other man in the office, it
always tired him very much. He also noticed an improvement in his temper. Having been so long in the
office, and knowing so much more about the business
than his fellow employees, he was frequently appealed
to for advice. These interruptions, before his sight became normal, were very annoying to him and often
caused him to lose his temper. Afterward, however, they
caused him no irritation whatever.

In another case, symptoms of insanity were relieved
when the vision became normal. The patient was a
physician who had been seen by many nerve and eye
specialists before he came to me, and who consulted me
at last, not because he had any faith in my methods, but
because nothing else seemed to be left for him to do.
He brought with him quite a collection of glasses prescribed by different men, no two of them being alike.
He had worn glasses, he told me, for many months at a
time without benefit, and then he had left them off and
had been apparently no worse. Outdoor life had also
failed to help him. On the advice of some prominent
neurologists he had even given up his practice for a
couple of years to spend the time upon a ranch, but the
vacation had done him no good.

I examined his eyes and found no organic defects and

no error of refraction. Yet his vision with each eye was only three-fourths of the normal and he suffered from double vision and all sorts of unpleasant symptoms. He used to see people standing on their heads and little devils dancing on the tops of the high buildings. He also had other illusions too numerous to be mentioned here. At night his sight was so bad that he had difficulty in finding his way about, and when walking along a country road he believed that he saw better when he turned his eyes far to one side and viewed the road with the side of the retina instead of with the center. At variable intervals, without warning and without loss of consciousness, he had attacks of blindness. These caused him great uneasiness, for he was a surgeon with a large and lucrative practice and he feared that he might have an attack while operating.

His memory was very poor. He could not remember the color of the eyes of any member of his family, although he had seen them all daily for years. Neither could he recall the color of his house, the number of rooms on the different floors or other details. The faces and names of patients and friends he recalled with difficulty or not at all.

His treatment proved to be very difficult, chiefly because he had an infinite number of erroneous ideas about physiological optics in general and his own case in particular, and insisted that all these should be discussed; while these discussions were going on he received no benefit. Every day for hours at a time over a long period he talked and argued. His logic was wonderful, apparently unanswerable, and yet utterly wrong.

His eccentric fixation was of such high degree that when he looked at a point forty-five degrees to one side of the big C on the Snellen test card he saw the letter just as black as when he looked directly at it. The strain to do this was terrific and produced much astigmatism; but the patient was unconscious of it and could not be convinced that there was anything abnormal in the symptom. If he saw the letter at all, he argued, he must see it as black as it really was, because he was not color-blind. Finally he became able to look away from one of the smaller letters on the card and see it worse than when he looked directly at it. It took eight or nine months to accomplish this, but when it had been done the patient said that it seemed as if a great burden had been lifted from his mind. He experienced a wonderful feeling of rest and relaxation throughout his whole body.

When asked to remember black with his eyes closed and covered he said he could not do so, and he saw every color but the black which one ought normally to see when the optic nerve is not subject to the stimulus of light. He had, however, been an enthusiastic football player at college, and he found at last that he could remember a black football. I asked him to imagine that this football had been thrown into the sea and that it was being carried outward by the tide, becoming constantly smaller but no less black. This he was able to do, and the strain floated with the football, until, by the time the latter had been reduced to the size of a period in a newspaper, it was entirely gone. The relief continued as long as he remembered the black spot, but as he could not remember it all the time, I suggested another method of gaining permanent relief. This was to make his sight voluntarily worse, a plan against which he protested with considerable emphasis.

"Good heavens!" he said. "Isn't my sight bad enough without making it worse?"

After a week of argument, however, he consented to try the method and the result was extremely satisfactory. After he had learned to see two or more lights where there was only one, by straining to see a point above the light while still trying to see the light as well as when looking directly at it, he became able to avoid the unconscious strain that had produced his double and multiple vision and was not troubled by these superfluous images any more. In a similar manner other illusions were prevented.

One of the last illusions to disappear was his belief that an effort was required to remember black. His logic on this point was overwhelming, but after many demonstrations he was convinced that no effort was required to let go, and when he realized this, both his vision and his mental condition immediately improved.

He finally became able to read 20/10 or more, and although more than fifty-five years of age, he also read diamond type at from six to twenty-four inches. His night blindness was relieved, his attacks of day blindness ceased, and he told me the color of the eyes of his wife and children. One day he said to me:

"Doctor, I thank you for what you have done for my sight, but no words can express the gratiude I feel for what you have done for my mind."

Some years later he called with his heart full of gratitude, because there had been no relapse.

From all these facts it will be seen that the problems of vision are far more intimately associated with the problems of education than we had supposed, and that they can by no means be solved by putting concave, or convex, or astigmatic lenses before the eyes of the children.

CHAPTER XXX

NORMAL SIGHT AND THE RELIEF OF PAIN FOR
SOLDIERS AND SAILORS

T HE Great War is over and among the millions
of brave men who laid down their lives in the
cruel conflict there were some who thought that
they were doing so that wars might be no more. But
the earth is still filled with wars and rumors of war, and
in the countries of the victorious Allies the spirit of militarism is rampant. In the United States we are being
urged to increase naval and military expenditure, and
there is a strong demand for universal military training.
Whether it is necessary for us to join in the competition
of armaments which resulted in the terrific convulsion
through which we have just passed is a question which
need not be entered into here; but if we are going to do
so, we may as well have soldiers and sailors with normal
sight; and if we attain this end we shall not have borne
the burdens of militarism and navalism altogether in
vain.

After the United States entered the recent war I had
the privilege of making it possible for many young men
who had been unable to meet the visual requirements
for admission to the army and navy, or to favorite
branches of these services, to gain normal vision; and
seeing no reason why such benefits should be confined
to the few, I supplied the Surgeon General of the Army
with a plan whereby, with far less trouble and expense
than was involved by the optical service upon which

we were then depending to make the worst of the enlisted eye-defectives available for service at the front, normal vision without glasses might have been insured to all soldiers and sailors. This plan was not acted upon, and I now present it, with some modifications, to the public, in the hope that enough people will see its military value to secure its adoption.

If we are to have universal military training, we shall find, as the nations of Europe have found, that it will be necessary to take measures to provide suitable material for such training. In Europe this necessity has resulted in extensive systems of child care, but in this book we are concerned only with the question of eyesight. In the first draft for the recent war, defective eyesight was the greatest single cause for rejection, while in later drafts it became one of three leading causes only because of an enormous lowering of an already low standard. Yet there is no impediment to the raising of an army which might be more easily removed. If we want our children to grow big enough to be soldiers, without losing most of their teeth and developing flat feet and crooked spines before they reach the military age, we shall have to make some arrangements, as every one of the advanced countries of Europe has done, for providing material as well as intellectual food in the schools. We shall have to employ school physicians on full time, and pay them enough to compensate men of eminence for the loss of private practice. We shall also have to see that the children are not sacrificed to the ignorance or poverty of their parents before they reach school age. But to preserve their eyesight it is only necessary to place Snellen test cards in every school classroom and see that the children read them every day. With this simple system of eye education beginning in the kindergarten and extending through the whole educational process up to the university and the professional school, it would soon be found that the young men of the country, on arrival at the military age, were practically free from eye defects.

But some years must elapse before this happy result can be achieved; and all eyes, moreover, no matter how good their vision, are benefited by the daily practice of the art of seeing, while by such practice those visual lapses to which every eye is subject, and which are particularly dangerous in military and naval operations, are either prevented or minimized. Therefore a system of eye education for training camps and the front should also be provided. For this purpose the method used in the schools could be modified.

Under conditions of actual warfare, or on the parade grounds of training camps, a Snellen test card might be impracticable, but there are other letters, or small objects, on the uniforms, on the guns, on the wagons, or elsewhere, which would serve the purpose equally well.

Letters or objects which require a vision of 20/20 should be selected by some one who has been taught what 20/20 means, and the men should be required to regard these letters or objects twice a day. After reading the letters they should be directed to cover their closed eyes with the palms of their hands to shut out all the light, and remember some color, preferably black, as well as they are able to see it, for half a minute. Then they should read the letters again and note any improvement in vision. The whole procedure would not take more than a minute. It should be made part of the regular drill, night and morning, and men with imperfect sight should be encouraged to repeat it as many times a day as convenient. They will need no urging: for imperfect vision is a bar to advancement and excludes from the favorite branch of the service, namely, aviation.

In each regiment every ten men should be under the supervision of one man who understands the method, and who must possess normal vision without glasses. He should carry a pocket test card, consisting of a few of the smaller letters, and should test the vision of the men at the beginning of the training, and thereafter at intervals of three months, reporting the results to the medical officer in charge.

Since errors of refraction are curable, no soldier should be allowed to wear glasses; but if the use of these aids to vision is permitted, the men wearing them should not be required to take part in the eye drills, as the method will do them no good under these conditions. When they see the benefits of eye education, however, they may wish to share them and will, no doubt, be willing to submit to the inconvenience resulting, temporarily, from going without their glasses.

In military colleges the same method could be used as in the schools; but a daily eye drill should also form part of the maneuvers on the parade ground, so that the students may be prepared to use it later in training camps or at the front.

To aviators, whether engaged in military or civilian operations, or whether they are flying merely for pleasure, eye education is of particular importance. Accidents to aviators, otherwise unaccountable, are easily explained when one understands how dependent the aviator is upon his eyesight, and how easily perfect vision may be lost amid the unaccustomed surroundings, the dangers and hardships of the upper air. It was formerly supposed that aviators maintained their equilibrium in the air by the aid of the internal ear; but it is now becoming evident from the testimony of aviators who have found themselves emerging from a cloud with one wing down, or even with their machines turned completely upside down, that equilibrium is maintained almost entirely, if not altogether, by the sense of sight.[1] If the aviator loses his sight, therefore, he is lost, and we have one of those "unaccountable" accidents which, during the war, were so unhappily common in the air service. All aviators, therefore, should make a daily practice of reading small, familiar letters, or observing other small, familiar objects, at a distance of ten feet or more. In addition, they should have a few small letters, or a single letter, on their machines, at a distance of five, ten, or more feet from their eyes, arrangements being made to illuminate them for night flying and fogs, and should read them frequently while in the air. This would greatly lessen the danger of visual lapses with their accompanying loss of equilibrium and judgment.

As has already been pointed out, eye education not only improves the sight, but affords a means by which pain, fatigue, the symptoms of disease and other discomforts can be relieved. For this latter purpose it is of the greatest value to soldiers and sailors; and if, during the recent war, they had only understood the simple and always available method of relieving pain by the aid of the memory, not only much suffering, but many deaths from the destructive effects of pain upon the body might have been prevented. A soldier in a flooded trench, if he can remember black perfectly, will know the temperature of

---

[1] Anderson: Lancet, March 16, 1918, p. 398; Hucks: Scientific American, October 6, 1917, p. 263.

the water, but will not suffer from cold. Under the same conditions he may succumb from weakness on the march, but will not feel fatigue. He may die of hemorrhage, but he will die painlessly. It will not be necessary to give him morphine to relieve his pain; and thus to the dangers of the battlefields will not be added the danger of returning to civil life under the handicap of a lifelong morphine habit.

This danger, there is reason to believe, assumed enormous proportions during the war. The Germans used a bullet which broke when it struck the bone and caused intense pain. The men often died of this pain before help arrived. When they were rescued the surgeons at once gave them morphine. A few hours later the injection was probably repeated. Then the drug was given less frequently, but in many cases it was not discontinued entirely while the man was in the hospital. A Red Cross surgeon at a meeting of the New York County Medical Society stated that he had been responsible for producing the morphine habit in thousands of soldiers, and that every physician at the front had done the same. By such a simple method as palming all this might have been prevented.

If we are going to have universal military and naval training, an essential part of that training should be the instruction of the prospective soldiers and sailors in the art of relieving their own pain; and in the event of war every one who goes to the front, in whatever capacity, from the generals and admirals down to the ambulance drivers, should understand palming. Everyone in the war zone, no matter how far behind the lines, may need this knowledge to relieve his own pain, and everyone may need it to relieve the pain of others.

CHAPTER XXXI

LETTERS FROM PATIENTS

The following letters have been selected almost at random from the author's mail-bag, and are only specimens of many more that are equally interesting. They are published because it was felt that the personal stories of patients, told in their own language, might be more interesting and helpful to many readers than the more formal presentation of the facts in the preceding chapters.

ARMY OFFICER CURES HIMSELF

AS noted in the chapter on "What Glasses Do to Us," the sight always improves when glasses are discarded, though this improvement may be so slight as not to be noticed. In a few unusual cases, the patients when freed from the handicap of a condition which compels them to keep their eyes continually under a strain, find out, in some way, how to avoid strain, and thus regain a greater or less degree of their normal visual power. The writer of the following letter was able, without any help from anyone, to discover and put into practice the main principles presented in this book, and thus became able to read without his glasses. He is an engineer, and at the time the letter was written was fifty-one years of age. He had worn glasses since 1896, first for astigmatism, getting stronger ones every couple of years, and then for astigmatism and presbyopia. At one time he asked his oculist and several opticians if the eyes could not be strengthened by exercises, so as to make glasses unnecessary, but they said: "No. Once started on glasses you must keep to them." When the war broke out he was very nearly disqualified for service in the Expeditionary Forces by his eyes, but managed to pass the required tests, after which he was ordered abroad as an officer in the Gas Service. While there he saw in the "Literary Digest" of May 2, 1918, a reference to my method of curing defective eyesight without glasses, and on May 11 he wrote to me in part as follows:

"At the front I found glasses a horrible nuisance, and they could not be worn with gas masks. After I had been about six months abroad I asked an officer of the Medical Corps about going without glasses. He said I was right in my ideas and told me to try it. The first week was awful, but I persisted and only wore glasses for reading and writing. I stopped smoking at the same time to make it easier on my nerves.

"I brought to France two pairs of bow spectacles and two extra lenses for repairs. I have just removed the extra piece for near vision from these extra lenses and had them mounted as pince-nez, with shur-on mounts, to use for reading and writing, so that the only glasses I now use are for astigmatism, the age lens being off. Three months ago I could not read ordinary head-line type in newspapers without glasses. To-day, with a good light, I can read ordinary book type, held at a distance of eighteen inches from my eyes. Since the first week in February, when I discarded my glasses, I have had no headaches, stomach trouble, or dizziness, and am in good health generally. My eyes are coming back, and I believe it is due to sticking it out. I ride considerably in automobiles and trams, and somehow the idea has crept into my mind that after every trip my eyes are stronger. This, I think, is due to the rapid changing of focus in viewing scenery going by so fast. Other men have tried this plan on my advice, but gave it up after two or three days. Yet, from what they say, I believe they were not so uncomfortable as I was for a week or ten days. I believe most people wear glasses because they 'coddle' their eyes."

The patient was right in thinking that the motor and tram rides improved his sight. The rapid motion compelled rapid shifting.

A TEACHER'S EXPERIENCES

It has frequently been pointed out in this book that imperfect vision is always associated with an abnormal state of the mind, and that when the vision improves the mental faculties improve also, to a greater or lesser degree. The following letter is a striking illustration of this fact. The writer, a teacher forty years of age, was first treated on March 28, 1919. She was wearing the following glasses: right eye, convex 0.75D.S. with convex 4.00D.C., 105 deg.; left eye, convex 0.75D.S. with convex 3.50D.C., 105 deg. On June 9, 1919, she wrote:

"I will tell you about my eyes, but first let me tell you other things. You were the first to unfold your theories to me, and I found them good immediately—that is, I was favorably impressed from the start. I did not take up the cure because other people recommended it, but because I was convinced: first, that you believed in your discovery yourself; second, that your theory of the cause of eye trouble was true. I don't know how I knew these two things, but I did. After a little conversation with you, you and your discovery both seemed to me to bear the ear-marks of the genuine article. As to the success of the method with myself I had a little doubt. You might cure others, but you might not be able to cure me. However, I took the plunge, and it has made a great change in me and my life.

"To begin with, I enjoy my sight. I love to look at things, to examine them in a leisurely, thorough way, much as a child examines things. I never realized it at the time, but it was irksome for me to look at things when I was wearing glasses, and I did as little of it as possible. The other day, going down on the Sandy Hook boat, I enjoyed a most wonderful sky without that hateful barrier of misted glasses, and I am positive I distinguished delicate shades of color that I never would have been able to see, even with clear glasses. Things seem to me now to have more form, more reality, than when I wore glasses. Looking into the mirror you see a solid representation on a flat surface, and the flat glass can't show you anything really solid. My eyeglasses, of course, never gave me this impression, but one curiously like it. I can see so clearly without them that it is like looking around corners without changing the position. I feel that I can almost do it.

"I very seldom have occasion to palm. Once in a great while I feel the necessity of it. The same with remembering a period. Nothing else is ever necessary. I seldom think of my eyes, but at times it is borne in upon me how much I do use and enjoy using them.

"My nerves are much better. I am more equable, have more poise, I am less shy. I never used to show that I was shy, or lacked confidence. I used to go ahead and do what was required, if not without hesitation; but it was hard. Now I find it easy. Glasses, or poor sight rather, made me self-conscious. It certainly is a great defect, and one people are sensitive to without realizing it. I mean the poor sight and the necessity for wearing glasses. I put on a pair of glasses the other day just for an experiment, and I found that they magnified things. My skin looked as if under a magnifying glass. Things seemed too near. The articles on my chiffonier looked so close I felt like pushing them away from me. The glasses I especially wanted to push away. They brought irritation at once. I took them off and felt peaceful. Things looked normal.

"From the beginning of the treatment I could use my eyes pretty well, but they used to tire. I remember making a large Liberty Loan poster two weeks after I took off my glasses, and I was amazed to find I could make the whole layout almost perfectly without a ruler, just as well as with my glasses. When I came to true it up with the ruler I found only the last row of letters a bit out of line at the very end. I couldn't have done better with glasses. However, this wasn't fine work. About the same time I sewed a hem at night in a black dress, using a fine needle. I suffered a little for this, but not much. I used to practice my exercises at that time, and palm faithfully. Now I don't have to practice, or palm; I feel no discomfort, and I am absolutely unsparing in my use of my eyes. I do everything I want to with them. I shirk nothing, pass up no opportunity of using them. From the first I did all my school work, read every notice, wrote all that was necessary, neglected nothing.

"Now to sum up the school end of it: I used to get headaches at the end of the month from adding columns of figures necessary to reports, etc. Now I do not get them. I used to get flustered when people came into my room. Now I do not; I welcome them. It is a pleasant change to feel this way. And—I suppose this is most important really, though I think of it last—I teach better. I know how to get at the mind and how to make the children see things in perspective. I gave a lesson on the horizontal cylinder recently, which, you know, is not a thrillingly interesting subject, and it was a remarkable lesson in its results and in the grip it got on every girl in the room, stupid or bright. What you have taught me makes me use the memory and imagination more, especially the latter, in teaching.

"To sum up the effect of being cured upon my own mind: I am more direct, more definite, less diffused, less vague. In short, I am conscious of being better centered. It is central fixation of the mind. I saw this in your latest paper, but I realized it long ago and knew what to call it."

A MENTAL TRANSITION

A man of forty-four who had worn glasses since the age of twenty was first seen on October 8, 1917, when he was suffering, not only from very imperfect sight, but from headache and discomfort. He was wearing for the right eye concave 5.00D.S. with concave 0.50D.C., 180 degrees, and for the left concave 2.50D.S. with concave 1.50D.C., 180 degrees. As his visits were not very frequent and he often went back to his glasses, his progress was slow. But his pain and discomfort were relieved very quickly, and almost from the beginning he had flashes of greatly improved and even of normal vision. This encouraged him to continue, and his progress, though slow, was steady. He has now gone without his glasses entirely for some months, and his nervous condition has improved as much as his sight. His wife was particularly impressed with the latter effect, and in December, 1919, she wrote:

"I have become very much interested in the thought of renewing my youth by becoming like a little child. The idea of the mental transition is not unfamiliar, but that this mental, or I should say spiritual, transition should produce a physical effect, which would lead to seeing clearly, is a sort of miracle very possible indeed, I should suppose, to those who have faith.

"In my husband's case, certainly some such miracle was wrought; for not only was he able to lay aside his spectacles after many years' constant use, and to see to read in almost any light, but I particularly noticed his serenity of mind after treatments. In this serenity he seemed able to do a great deal of work efficiently, and not under the high nervous pressure whose after-effect is the devastating scattering of forces.

"It did not occur to me for a long time that perhaps your treatment was quieting his nerves. But I think now that the quiet periods of relaxation, two or three times a day, during which he practiced with the letter card, must have had a very beneficial effect. He is so enthusiastic by nature, and his nerves are so easily stimulated, that for years he used to overdo periodically. Of course, his greatly improved eyesight and the relief from the former strain must have been a large factor in this improvement. But I am inclined to think that the intervals of quiet and peace were wonderfully beneficial, and why shouldn't they be? We are living on stimulants, physical stimulants, mental stimulants of all kinds. The minute these stop we feel we are merely existing, and yet, if we retain any of the normality of our youth, do you not think that we respond very happily to natural simple things?"

RELIEF AFTER TWENTY-FIVE YEARS

While many persons are benefited by the accepted methods of treating defects of vision, there is a minority of cases, known to every eye specialist, which gets little or no help from them. These patients sometimes give up the search for relief in despair, and sometimes continue it with surprising pertinacity, never being able to abandon the belief, in spite of the testimony of experience, that somewhere in the world there must be some one with sufficient skill to fit them with the right glasses. The rapidity with which these patients respond to treatment by relaxation is often very dramatic, and affords a startling illustration of the superiority of this method to treatment by glasses and muscle-cutting. In the following case relaxation did in twenty-four hours what the old methods, as practiced by a succession of eminent specialists, could not do in twenty-five years.

The patient was a man of forty-nine, and his imperfect sight was accompanied by continual pain and misery, culminating twenty years before I saw him, in a complete nervous breakdown. As he was a writer, dependent upon his pen for a living, his condition was a serious economic handicap, and he consulted many specialists in the vain hope of obtaining relief. Glasses did little either to improve his sight, or to relieve his discomfort, and the eye specialists talked vaguely about disease of the optic nerve and brain as a possible cause of his troubles. The nerve specialists, however, were unable to do anything to relieve him. One specialist diagnosed his case as muscular, and gave him prisms, which helped him a little.

Later, the same specialist, finding that all of the apparent muscular trouble was not corrected by glasses, cut the external muscles of both eyes. This also brought some relief, but not much. At the age of twenty-nine the patient suffered the nervous breakdown already mentioned. For this he was treated unsuccessfully by various specialists, and for nine years he was compelled to live out of doors. This life, although it benefited him, failed to restore his health, and when he came to me on September 13, 1919, he was still suffering from neurasthenia. His distant vision was less than 20/40, and could not be improved by glasses. He was able to read with glasses, but could not do so without discomfort. I could find no symptom of disease of the brain or of the interior of the eye. When he tried to palm he saw grey and yellow instead of black; but he was able to rest his eyes simply by closing them, and by this means alone he became able, in twenty-four hours, to read diamond type and to make out most of the letters on the twenty line of the test card at twenty feet. At the same time his discomfort was materially relieved. He was under treatment for about six weeks, and on October 25 he wrote as follows:

"I saw you last on October 6, and at the end of the week, the 11th, I started off on a ten-day motor trip as one of the officials of the Cavalry Endurance Test for horses. The last touch of eyestrain which affected me nervously at all I experienced on the 8th and 9th. On the trip, though I averaged but five hours' sleep, rode all day in an open motor without goggles and wrote reports at night by bad lights, I had no trouble. After the third day the universal slow swing seemed to establish itself, and I have never had a moment's discomfort since. I stood fatigue and excitement better than I have ever done, and went with less sleep. My practicing on the trip was necessarily somewhat curtailed, yet there was noticeable improvement in my vision. Since returning I have spent a couple of hours a day in practice, and have at the same time done a lot of writing.

"Yesterday, the 24th, I made a test with diamond type, and found that after twenty minutes' practice I could get the lines distinct, and make out the capital letters and bits of the text at a scant three inches. At seven I could read it readily, though I could not see it perfectly. This was by an average daylight—no sun. In a good daylight I can read the newspaper almost perfectly at a normal reading distance, say fifteen inches.

"I feel now that I am really out of the woods. I have done night work without suffering for it, a thing I have not done in twenty-five years, and I have worked steadily for more hours than I have been able to work at a time since my breakdown in 1899, all without sense of strain or nervous fatigue. You can imagine my gratitude to you. Not only for my own sake, but for yours, I shall leave no stone unturned to make the cure complete and get back the child eyes which seem perfectly possible in the light of the progress I have made in eight weeks."

SEEKING A MYOPIA CURE

In spite of the emphasis with which the medical profession denies the possibility of curing errors of refraction, there are many lay persons who refuse to believe that they are incurable. The author of the following statement represents a considerable class, and was remarkable only in the persistency with which he searched for relief. He was first seen on June 27, 1919, at which time he was thirty-two years of age. He was wearing concave 2.50D.S. for each eye, and his vision in each eye was 20/100—. After he had obtained almost normal vision he wrote the following account of his experiences for "Better Eyesight":

"When the 'Lusitania' was sunk I knew that the United States was going to get into trouble, and I wanted to be in a position to join the Army. But I was suffering from a high degree of myopia, and I knew they wouldn't take me with glasses. Later on they took almost anyone who wasn't blind, but at that time I couldn't possibly have measured up to the standard. So I began to look about for a cure. I tried osteopathy, but didn't go very far with it. I asked the optician who had been fitting me with glasses for advice, but he said that myopia was incurable. I dismissed the matter for a time, but I didn't stop thinking about it. I am a farmer, and I knew from the experience of outdoor life that health is the normal condition of living beings. I knew that when health is lost it can often be regained. I knew that when I first tried to lift a barrel of apples onto a wagon I could not do so, but that after a little practice I became able to do it easily, and I did not see why, if one part of the body could be strengthened by exercise, others could not be strengthened also. I could remember a time when I was not myopic, and it seemed to me that if a normal eye could become myopic, it ought to be possible for a myopic eye to regain normality. After a while I went back to the optician and told him that I was convinced that there must be some cure for my condition. He replied that this was quite impossible, as everyone knew that myopia was incurable. The assurance with which he made this statement had an effect upon me quite the opposite of what he intended, for when he said that the cure of myopia was impossible I knew that it was not, and I resolved never to give up the search for a cure until I found it. Shortly after I had the good fortune to hear of Dr. Bates, and lost no time in going to see him. At the first visit I was able, just by closing and resting my eyes, to improve my sight considerably for the Snellen test card, and after a few months of intermittent treatment I became able to read 20/10—in flashes. I am still improving, and when I can see a little better I mean to go back to that optician and tell him what I think of his ophthalmological learning."

FACTS VERSUS THEORIES

Reading fine print is commonly supposed to be an extremely dangerous practice, and reading print of any kind upon a moving vehicle is thought to be even worse. Looking away to the distance, however, and not seeing anything in particular is believed to be very beneficial to the eyes. In the light of these superstitions, the facts contained in the following letter are particularly interesting:

"On reaching home Monday morning I was surprised and pleased at the comments of my family regarding the appearance of my eyes. They all thought they looked so much brighter and rested, and that after two days of railroading. I didn't spare my eyes in the least on the way home. I read magazines and newspapers, looked at the scenery; in fact, used my eyes all the time. My sight for the near-point is splendid. Can read for hours without tiring my eyes. . . . I went downtown today and my eyes were very tired when I got home. The fine print on the card [diamond type] helps me so.. . . I would like to have your little Bible [a photographic reduction of the Bible with type much smaller than diamond]. I'm sure the very fine print has a soothing effect on one's eyes, regardless of what my previous ideas on the subject were."

It will be observed that the eyes of this patient were not tired by her two days' railroad journey, during which she read constantly; they were not tired by hours of reading after her return; they were rested by reading extremely fine print; but they were very much tired by a trip downtown during which they were not called upon to focus upon small objects. Later a leaf from the Bible was sent to her, and she wrote:

"The effect even of the first effort to read it was wonderful. If you will believe it, I haven't been troubled having my eyes feel 'crossed' since, and while my actual vision does not seem to be any better, my eyes feel a great deal better."

CURED WITHOUT PERSONAL ASSISTANCE

I am constantly hearing of patients who have been able to improve their sight by the aid of information contained in my publications, without personal assistance. The writer of the following letter, a physician, is a remarkable example of these cases, as he was able not only to cure himself, but to relieve some very serious cases of defective vision among his patients.

"I first tried central fixation on myself and had marvelous results. I threw away my glasses and can now see better than I have ever done. I read very fine type (smaller than newspaper type) at a distance of six inches from the eyes, and can run it out at full arm's length and still read it without blurring the type.

"I have instructed some of my patients in your

methods, and all are getting results. One case who has a partial cataract of the left eye could not see anything on the Snellen test card at twenty feet, and could see the letters only faintly at ten feet. Now she can read 20/10 with both eyes together, and also with each eye separately; but the left eye seems, as she says, to be looking through a little fog. I could cite many other cases that have been benefited by central fixation, but this one is the most interesting to me."

CHAPTER XXXII

REASON AND AUTHORITY

SOME one—perhaps it was Bacon—has said: "You cannot by reasoning correct a man of ill opinion which by reasoning he never acquired." He might have gone a step further and stated that neither by reasoning, nor by actual demonstration of the facts, can you convince some people that an opinion which they have accepted on authority is wrong.

A man whose name I do not care to mention, a professor of ophthalmology, and a writer of books well known in this country and in Europe, saw me perform the experiment illustrated on Page 40, an experiment which, according to others who witnessed it, demonstrates beyond any possibility of error that the lens is not a factor in accommodation. At each step of the operation he testified to the facts; yet at the conclusion he preferred to discredit the evidence of his senses rather than accept the only conclusion that these facts admitted.

First he examined the eye of the animal to be experimented upon, with the retinoscope, and found it normal, and the fact was written down. Then the eye was stimulated with electricity, and he testified that it accommodated. This was also written down. I now divided the superior oblique muscle, and the eye was again stimulated with electricity. The doctor observed the eye with the retinoscope when this was being done and said: "You failed to produce accommodation." This fact, too, was written down. The doctor now used the electrode himself, but again failed to observe accommodation, and these facts were written down. I now sewed the cut ends of the muscle together, and once more stimulated the eye with electricity. The doctor said, "Now you have succeeded in producing accommodation," and this was written down. I now asked:

"Do you think that superior oblique had anything to do with producing accommodation?"

"Certainly not," he replied.

"Why?" I asked.

"Well," he said, "I have only the testimony of the retinoscope; I am getting on in years, and I don't feel that confidence in my ability to use the retinoscope that I once had. I would rather you wouldn't quote me on this."

While the operation was in progress, however, he gave no indication whatever of doubting his ability to use the retinoscope. He was very positive, in fact, that I had failed to produce accommodation after the cutting of the oblique muscle, and his tone suggested that he considered the failure ignominious. It was only after he found himself in a logical trap, with no way out except by discrediting his own observations, that he appeared to have any doubts as to their value.

Patients whom I have cured of various errors of refraction have frequently returned to specialists who had prescribed glasses for them, and, by reading fine print and the Snellen test card with normal vision, have demonstrated the fact that they were cured, without in any way shaking the faith of these practitioners in the doctrine that such cures are impossible.

The patient with progressive myopia whose case was mentioned in Chapter XV returned after her cure to the specialist who had prescribed her glasses, and who had said not only that there was no hope of improvement, but that the condition would probably progress until it ended in blindness, to tell him the good news which, as an old friend of her family, she felt he had a right to hear. But while he was unable to deny that her vision was, in fact, normal without glasses, he said it was impossible that she should have been cured of myopia, because myopia was incurable. How he reconciled this statement with his former patient's condition he was unable to make clear to her.

A lady with compound myopic astigmatism suffered from almost constant headaches which were very much worse when she took her glasses off. The theatre and the movies caused her so much discomfort that she feared to indulge in these recreations. She was told to take off her glasses and advised, among other things, to go to the movies; to look first at the corner of the screen, then off to the dark, then back to the screen a little nearer to the center, and so forth. She did so, and soon became able to look directly at the pictures without discomfort. After that nothing troubled her. One day she called on her former ophthalmological adviser, in the company of a friend who wanted to have her glasses changed, and told him of her cure. The facts seemed to make no impression on him whatever. He only laughed and said, "I guess Dr. Bates is more popular with you than I am."

Sometimes patients themselves, after they are cured, allow themselves to be convinced that it was impossible that such a thing could have happened, and go back to their glasses. This happened in the case of a patient already mentioned in the chapter on "Presbyopia," who was cured in fifteen minutes by the aid of his imagination. He was very grateful for a time, and then he began to talk to eye specialists whom he knew and straightway grew skeptical as to the value of what I had done for him.

One day I met him at the home of a mutual friend, and in the presence of a number of other people he accused me of having hypnotized him, adding that to hypnotize a patient without his knowledge or consent was to do him a grievous wrong. Some of the listeners protested that whether I had hypnotized him or not, I had not only done him no harm but had greatly benefited him, and he ought to forgive me. He was unable, however, to take this view of the matter. Later he called on a prominent eye specialist who told him that the presbyopia and astigmatism from which he had suffered were incurable, and that if he persisted in going without his glasses he might do himself great harm. The fact that his sight was perfect for the distance and the near-point without glasses had no effect upon the specialist, and the patient allowed himself to be frightened into disregarding it also. He went back to his glasses, and so far as I know has been wearing them ever since. The story obtained wide publicity, for the man had a large circle of friends and acquaintances; and if I had destroyed his sight I could scarcely have suffered more than I did for curing him.

Fifteen or twenty years ago the specialist mentioned in the foregoing story read a paper on cataract at a meeting of the ophthalmological section of the American Medical Association in Atlantic City, and asserted that anyone who said that cataract could be cured without the knife was a quack. At that time I was assistant surgeon at the New York Eye and Ear Infirmary, and it happened that I had been collecting statistics of the spontaneous cure of cataract at the request of the executive surgeon of this institution, Dr. Henry G. Noyes, Professor of Ophthalmology at the Bellevue Hospital Medical School. As a result of my inquiry, I had secured records of a large num-

ber of cases which had recovered, not only without the
knife, but without any treatment at all.   I also had records of cases which I had sent to Dr. James E. Kelly of
New York and which he had cured, largely by hygienic
methods.   Dr. Kelly is not a quack, and at that time was
Professor of Anatomy in the New York Post Graduate
Medical School and Hospital and attending surgeon to a
large city hospital.   In the five minutes allotted to those
who wished to discuss the paper, I was able to tell the
audience enough about these cases to make them want
to hear more.   My time was, therefore, extended, first to
half an hour and then to an hour.   Later both Dr. Kelly
and myself received many letters from men in different
parts of the country who had tried his treatment with
success.   The man who wrote the paper had blundered,
but he did not lose any prestige because of my attack,
with facts upon his theories.   He is still a prominent and
honored ophthalmologist, and in his latest book he gives
no hint of having ever heard of any successful method of
treating cataract other than by operation.   He was not
convinced by my record of spontaneous cures, nor by Dr.
Kelly's record of cures by treatment; and while a few
men were sufficiently impressed to try the treatment
recommended, and while they obtained satisfactory results, the facts made no impression upon the profession
as a whole, and did not modify the teaching of the
schools.   That spontaneous cures of cataract do sometimes occur cannot be denied; but they are supposed to
be very rare, and any one who suggests that the condition can be cured by treatment still exposes himself to
the suspicion of being a quack.

Between 1886 and 1891 I was a lecturer at the Post-
Graduate Hospital and Medical School.   The head of the
institution was Dr. D. B. St. John Roosa.   He was the

author of many books, and was honored and respected by the whole medical profession. At the school they had got the habit of putting glasses on the nearsighted doctors, and I had got the habit of curing them without glasses. It was naturally annoying to a man who had put glasses on a student to have him appear at a lecture without them and say that Dr. Bates had cured him. Dr. Roosa found it particularly annoying, and the trouble reached a climax one evening at the annual banquet of the faculty when, in the presence of one hundred and fifty doctors, he suddenly poured out the vials of his wrath upon my head. He said that I was injuring the reputation of the Post Graduate by claiming to cure myopia. Every one knew that Donders said it was incurable, and I had no right to claim that I knew more than Donders. I reminded him that some of the men I had cured had been fitted with glasses by himself. He replied that if he had said they had myopia he had made a mistake. I suggested further investigation. "Fit some more doctors with glasses for myopia," I said, "and I will cure them. It is easy for you to examine them afterwards and see if the cure is genuine." This method did not appeal to him, however. He repeated that it was impossible to cure myopia, and to prove that it was impossible he expelled me from the Post Graduate, even the privilege of resignation being denied to me.

The fact is that, except in rare cases, man is not a reasoning being. He is dominated by authority, and when the facts are not in accord with the view imposed by authority, so much the worse for the facts. They may, and indeed must, win in the long run; but in the meantime the world gropes needlessly in darkness and endures much suffering that might have been avoided.

50 FEET

C

30 FEET

R B

20 FEET

T F P

15 FEET

5 C G O

10 FEET

4 K B E R

5 FEET

3 V Y F P T

4 FEET

2 Q C O G D □ C

3 FEET`

R Z 3 B 8 S H K F O

2 FEET

F T Y V P E C □ O B R K 5 6

310

SUGGESTIONS TO PATIENTS
The Use of the Snellen Test Card

1—Every home should have a test card.

2—It is best to place the card permanently on the wall in a good light.

3—Each member of the family or household read the card every day.

4—It takes only a minute to test the sight with the card. If you spend five minutes in the morning practicing with the card, it will be a great help during the day.

5—Place yourself ten feet from the card and read as far as you can without effort or strain. Over each line of letters are small figures indicating the distance. Over the big C at the top is the figure 50. The big C, therefore, should be read at a distance of 50 feet.

6—If you can only see the fifth line, notice that the last letter on that line is an R. Now close your eyes, cover them with the palms of the hands and remember the R. If you will remember that the left side is straight, the right side partly curved and the bottom open, you will get a good mental picture of the R with your eyes closed. This mental picture will help you to see the letter directly underneath the R, which is a T.

7—Shifting is good to stop the stare. If you stare at the letter T, you will notice that all the letters on that line begin to blur. It is beneficial to close your eyes quickly after you see the T, open them, and shift to the first figure on that line, which is a 3. Then close your eyes and remember the 3. You will become able to read all the letters on that line by closing your eyes for each letter.

8—Keep a record of each test in order to note your progress from day to day.

311

CHAPTER XXXIII

HOW TO DEMONSTRATE THE FUNDAMENTAL
PRINCIPLES OF TREATMENT

THE object of all the methods used in the treatment of imperfect sight without glasses is to secure rest or relaxation, of the mind first and then of the eyes. Rest always improves the vision. Effort always lowers it. Persons who wish to improve their vision should begin by demonstrating these facts.

To demonstrate the strain lowers the vision, think of something disagreeable, some physical discomfort, or something seen imperfectly. When the eyes are opened, it will be found that the vision has been lowered. Also stare at one part of a letter on the test card, or try to see the whole letter all alike at one time. This invariably lowers the vision, and may cause the letters to disappear. Another symptom of strain is a twitching of the eyelids which can be seen by an observer and felt by the patient with the fingers. This can usually be corrected if the period of rest is long enough. Many persons fail to secure a temporary improvement of vision by closing their eyes, because they do not keep them closed long enough. Children will seldom do this unless a grown person stands by and encourages them. Many adults also require supervision.

CLOSING THE EYES

The simplest way to rest the eyes is to close them for a longer or shorter period and think about something agreeable. This is always the first thing that I tell patients to do and there are very few who are not benefited by it temporarily.

PALMING

A still greater degree of rest can be obtained by closing and covering the eyes so as to exclude all the light. The mere exclusion of the impression of sight is often sufficient to produce a large measure of relaxation. In other cases the strain is increased. As a rule, successful palming involves a knowledge of various other means of obtaining relaxation. The mere covering and closing of the eyes is useless unless at the same time mental rest is obtained. When a patient palms perfectly he sees a field so black that it is impossible to remember, imagine, or see anything blacker, and when able to do this he is cured. It should be borne in mind, however, that the patient's judgment of what is a perfect black is not to be depended upon.

THE LONG SWING

Demonstrate—That the long swing not only improves the vision, but also relieves or cures pain, discomfort and fatigue.

Stand with the feet about one foot apart, facing squarely one side of the room. Lift the left heel a short distance from the floor while turning the shoulders, head, and eyes to the right, until the line of the shoulders is parallel with the wall. Now turn the body to the left after placing the left heel upon the floor and raising the right heel. Alternate looking from the right wall to the left wall, being careful to move the head and eyes with the movement of the shoulders. When practiced easily, continuously, without effort and without paying any attention to moving objects, one soon becomes conscious that the long swing relaxes the tension of the muscles and nerves.

Stationary objects move with varying degrees of rapidity. Objects located almost directly in front of you appear to move with express train speed and should be very much blurred. It is very important to make no attempt to see clearly objects which seem to be moving very rapidly.

The long swing seems to help patients who suffer from eyestrain during sleep. By practicing the long swing fifty times or more just before retiring and just after rising in the morning, eyestrain during sleep has been prevented or relieved. It is remarkable how quickly the long swing relieves or prevents pain. I know of no other procedure which can compare with it. The long swing has relieved the pain of facial neuralgia after operative measures had failed. Some patients who have suffered from continuous pain in various parts of the body have been relieved by the long swing, at first temporarily, but by repetition the relief has become more permanent. Hay fever, asthma, sea-sickness, palpitation of the heart, coughs, acute and chronic colds are usually relieved by the long swing.

MEMORY

When the sight is normal the mind is always perfectly at rest, and when the memory is perfect the mind is also at rest. Therefore it is possible to improve the sight by the use of the memory. Anything the patient finds it agreeable to remember is a rest to the mind, but for purposes of practice a small black object, such as a period or a letter of fine print, is usually most convenient. The most favorable condition for the exercise of the memory is, usually, with the eyes closed and covered, but by practice it becomes possible to remember equally well with the eyes open. When patients are able, with their eyes closed and covered, to remember perfectly a letter of fine print, it appears, just as it would if they were looking at it with the bodily eyes, to have a slight movement, while the openings appear whiter than the rest of the background. If they are not able to remember it, they are told to shift consciously from one side of the letter to another and to consciously imagine the opening whiter than the rest of the background. When they do this, the letter usually appears to move in a direction contrary to that of the imagined movement of the eye, and they are able to remember it indefinitely. If, on the contrary, they try to fix the attention on one part of the letter, or to think of two or more parts at one time, it soon disappears, demonstrating that it is impossible to think of one point continuously, or to think of two or more points perfectly at one time, just as it is impossible to look at a point continuously, or to see two points perfectly at the same time. Persons with no visual memory are always under a great strain and often suffer from pain and fatigue with no apparent cause. As soon as they become able to form mental pictures, either with the eyes closed or open, their pain and fatigue are relieved.

IMAGINATION

Imagination is closely allied to memory, for we can imagine only as well as we remember, and in the treatment of imperfect sight the two can scarcely be separated. Vision is largely a matter of imagination and memory. And since both imagination and memory are impossible without perfect relaxation, the cultivation of these faculties not only improves the interpretation of the pictures on the retina, but improves the pictures themselves. When you imagine that you see a letter on the test card you actually do see it, because it is impossible to relax and imagine the letter perfectly, and, at the same time, strain and see it imperfectly. The following method of using the imagination has produced quick results in many cases. The patient is asked to look at the largest letter on the test card at the near-point, and is usually able to observe that a small area, about a square inch, appears blacker than the rest, and that when the part of the letter seen worst is covered, part of the exposed area seems blacker than the remainder. When the part seen worst is again covered, the area of maximum blackness is still further reduced. When the part seen best has been reduced to about the size of a letter on the bottom line, the patient is asked to imagine that such a letter occupies this area and is blacker than the rest of the letter. Then he is asked to look at a letter on the bottom line and imagine that it is blacker than the largest letter. Many are able to do this, and at once become able to see the letters on the bottom line.

FLASHING

Since it is effort that spoils the sight, many persons with imperfect sight are able, after a period of rest, to look at an object for a fraction of a second. If the eyes are closed before the habit of strain reasserts itself permanent relaxation is sometimes very quickly obtained. This practice I have called flashing, and many persons are helped by it who are unable to improve their sight by other means. The eyes are rested for a few minutes, by closing or palming, and then a letter on the test card, or a letter of fine print, if the trouble is with near vision, is regarded for a fraction of a second. Then the eyes are immediately closed and the process repeated.

READING FAMILIAR LETTERS

The eye always strains to see unfamiliar objects, and is always relaxed to a greater or less degree by looking at familiar objects. Therefore the reading every day of small familiar letters at the greatest distance at which they can be seen is a rest to the eye, and is sufficient to cure children under twelve who have not worn glasses, as well as some older children, and adults with minor defects of vision.

CENTRAL FIXATION

When the vision is normal the eye sees one part of everything it looks at best and every other part worse in proportion as it is removed from the point of maximum vision. When the vision is imperfect it is invariably found that the eye is trying to see a considerable part of its field of vision equally well at one time. This is a great strain upon the eye and mind, as anyone whose sight is approximately normal can demonstrate by trying to see an appreciable area all alike at one time. At the near-point the attempt to see an area even a quarter of an inch in diameter in this way will produce discomfort and pain. Anything which rests the eye tends to restore the normal power of central fixation. It can also be regained by conscious practice, and this is sometimes the quickest and easiest way to improve the sight. When the patient becomes conscious that he sees one part of his field of vision better than the rest, it usually becomes possible for him to reduce the area seen best. If he looks from the bottom of the 200 letter to the top, for instance, and sees the part not directly regarded worse than the part fixed, he may become able to do the same with the next line of letters, and thus he may become able to go down the card until he can look from the top to the bottom of the letters on the bottom line and see the part not directly regarded worse. In that case he will be able to read the letters. Since small objects cannot be seen without central fixation, the reading of fine print, when it can be done, is one of the best of visual exercises, and the dimmer the light in which it can be read and the closer to the eye it can be held the better.

THE EFFECT OF LIGHT UPON THE EYES AND SUN TREATMENT

Although the eyes were made to react to the light, a very general fear of the effect of this element upon the organs of vision is entertained both by the medical profession and by the laity. Persons with normal sight have been able to look at the sun for a short length of time, without any discomfort or loss of vision. Immediately afterward they were able to read the Snellen test card with improved vision, their sight having become better than what is ordinarily considered normal. Some persons with normal sight do suffer discomfort and loss of vision when they look at the sun; but in such cases the retinoscope always indicates an error of refraction, showing that this condition is due, not to the light, but to strain. It has been my experience that all persons who wear dark glasses sooner or later develop inflammation of their eyes. The human eye needs the light in order to maintain its efficiency. The use of eye-shades and protections of all kinds from the light is injurious to the eyes. Sunlight is as necessary to normal eyes as is rest and relaxation. If it is possible, start the day by exposing the closed eyes to the sun. Just a few minutes at a time will help. Get accustomed to the strong light of the sun by letting it shine on your closed eyelids. It is good to move the head slightly from side to side while doing this, in order to prevent straining. One cannot get too much sun treatment

BRAIN TENSION

The brain has many nerves. Part of these nerves are called ganglion cells and originate in some particular part of the brain. Each has a function of its own. They are connected with other ganglion cells and with the aid of nerve fibres are connected with others located in various parts of the brain as well as in the spinal cord, the eye, the ear, the nerves of smell, taste, and the nerves of touch. The function of each ganglion cell of the brain is different from that of all others. When the ganglion cells are healthy, they function in a normal manner.

The retina of the eye contains numerous ganglion cells which regulate special things such as normal vision, normal memory, normal imagination and they do this with a control more or less accurate of other ganglion cells of the whole body. The retina has a similar structure to parts of the brain. It is connected to the brain by the optic nerve.

Many nerves from the ganglion cells of the retina carry conscious and unconscious control of other ganglion cells which are connected to other parts of the body.

When the ganglion cells are diseased or at fault, the functions of all parts of the body are not normally maintained. In all cases of imperfect sight, it has been repeatedly demonstrated that the ganglion cells and nerves of the brain are under a strain. When this strain is corrected by treatment, the functions of the ganglion and other cells become normal. The importance of the mental treatment cannot be over-estimated.

A study of the facts has demonstrated that a disease of some ganglion in any part of the body occurs in a similar ganglion in the brain.

Brain tension of one or more nerves always means disease of the nerve ganglia. Treatment of the mind with the aid of the sight, memory and imagination has cured many cases of imperfect sight without other treatment.

Doctor William H. Bates—An Appreciation
by Dr. Daniel A. Poling

I never knew Doctor Bates when physically he was a well man. But even in the comparatively short time of our acquaintance and friendship I never knew him when he was not a true gentleman and a veritable genius in thinking thoughts and doing deeds for others. In his profession he was a distinguished pioneer; his discoveries should give him a place among the benefactors of the race. All about me and in my own home are those to whom he has ministered. To the ends of the earth are men, women, and little children who think of him with gratitude because of pain relieved and sight restored. His welcome to the Father's House will be in the words of the immortal paean—"Well done, good and faithful servant." By every test that I know, since I have known him, Doctor Bates was a Christian. One of his favorite texts was, "As a man thinketh in his heart so is he." The good Doctor had many and long thoughts of others and always his longest, tenderest thoughts were for Mrs. Emily A. Bates who has been his comrade in a great service.

With those who have the Christian's hope, weeping endures but for the night. We sorrow but not as those who are without the promise of glad reunion. Today we lift our eyes to the hills from whence cometh our strength—the hills of God's country where dreams come true, where unfinished tasks are completed and where life with love, enters fulfillment.

Signed Daniel A. Poling

INDEX

Accommodation, 10, 26 (see also "Aphakia," "Myopia," "Presbyopia")
  Arlt on, 29
  Author on, 38, 54, 69
  Brücke on, 29
  Cohn on, 29
  Cramer on, 25
  Davis on, 33
  Descartes on, 24
  Donders on, 24, 29, 32, 38, 210, 211
  Duane on, 211
  Förster on, 32
  Fuchs on, 211
  von Graefe on, 32
  Helmholtz on, 24, 26, 32
  Hensen on, 29
  Holmes on, 212
  Huxley on, 29
  Jackson on, 211
  Kepler on, 23
  Landolt on, 26
  Langenbeck on, 24
  Loring on, 33
  Roosa on, 210
  Sanson on, 29
  Scheiner on, 24
  Tscherning on, 27
  de Schweinitz on, 36, 211
  Völckers on, 29
  Young on, 24, 30
Ainus, 16
Amblyopia, 111, 113 (see also "Squint")
Anisometropes, 256
Aphakia, 32, 47, 95, 96
Arlt, 29
  portrait. frontispiece

Armati, v, 81
Astigmatism, 12, 70, 149, 251
  prevention, 251, 265
  production, 12, 36, 39, 42, 43, 45, 89, 266, 282
  treatment, 229, 234, 273, 306 (see also "Refraction, errors of, treatment")
Atropine, 43, 48, 50, 69, 228, 234
Aviators, 287

Barrington, 256
Bell, 184
Brücke, 29

Camera, 13, 114, 149
Cataract, 89, 111, 214, 220
  treatment, 121, 134, 158, 272, 307
Central fixation, 114, 281
Christian Scientists, 209
Cohn, 29, 78, 251, 252, 253, 254
Colds, 208
Conjunctiva, 111, 118, 122
Cornea, 12, 36, 122 (see also "Images, on cornea")
Correspondence treatment, 246
Coughs, 208
Cramer, 25

Darkness, 189
Davis, 33
Descartes, 24
Donders, 23, 24, 25, 29, 32, 38, 210, 211, 222, 223
Dresslar, 190
Duane, 211, 225

Eccentric fixation (see "Central fixation")
Emmetropia, 11, 93
Eversbusch, 222, 252
Eye, 11, 13
    evolution of, 1
    muscles of, 38, 44
    retina of, 114
    unable to fix a point, 159

Fabre, 102
Face-rests, 253, 254
Faith Curists, 209
Förster, 32
Fovea, 114
Fox, 256
Fuchs, 211, 222, 225

Gislason, 227
Glasses, v, 8, 81, 181, 219
Glaucoma, 111, 220
    treatment, 121, 133, 208
Gould, 4
von Graefe, 32

Hansen-Grut, 222
Hay fever, 208
Helmholtz, 24, 26, 32, 36, 38
    portrait, 31
Helpful Suggestions, 312
Hensen, 29
Holmes, 212
Home treatment, 242
Huxley, 29
Hypermetropia, 10, 222, 251, 266
    prevention, 251, 266
    production, 14, 39, 42, 53, 63, 65, 66, 75, 89, 266
    treatment, 229, 234, 273
        (see also "Refraction, errors of, treatment")

Illusions,
    of imperfect sight, 148, 172, 219, 280, 282
    of normal sight, 138, 172, 180

Images, 24, 54
    on cornea, 24, 54, 59, 60, 64, 66, 68
    on iris, 59, 63, 65
    on lens (back of), 24, 54, 62, 67
    on lens (front of), 24, 54
    on sclera, 59, 62, 63, 64
Imagination, 148, 165, 217
Indians, 2, 15, 256
Insanity, 280
Iritis, 121, 122

Jackson, 211
Johnson, 37
Jupiter, moons of, 103, 121, 275
Just, 254

Kelly, 308
Kepler, 23

Lancaster, 83
Landolt, 23, 26, 86
Langenbeck, 24
Lawson, 255
Lens (see "Accommodation," "Cataract," "I m a g e s," "Presbyopia")
Light, 78, 123, 183, 253, 261
Loring, 33

Macaulay, 275
Macula, 114
Memory, 126, 136, 151, 202, 274
Military training, 284
Mind, 89, 106, 115, 148, 196, 274, 295 (see also "Memory")
Montessori, 106
Moros, 6
Morphine, 289
Motais, 256
Moving pictures, 108, 161, 192
Muscae volitantes, 176, 236
Muscle, ciliary, 11, 29, 75, 85, 211, 215 (see also "Atropine")
Muscles, external, 32, 37, 38, 89

Myopia, 8, 10, 222 (see also
   "Accommodation")
   Barrington on, 256
   Cohn on, 251, 252, 253, 254
   Donders on, 309
   Eversbusch on, 252
   Fox on, 256
   Just on, 254
   Lawson on, 255
   Motais on, 256
   Pearson on, 256
   prevention, 8, 39, 251, 259
   production, 2, 11, 14, 63,
    65, 75, 89, 109, 257
   Risley on, 253
   Roosa on, 308
   Sidler-Huguenin on, 8, 82,
    256
   Steiger on, 256
   treatment, 8, 82, 120, 141,
    157, 158, 170, 251, 259,
    271, 299 (see also "Re-
    fraction, errors of, treat-
    ment")
   Tscherning on, 252

Neuralgia, 207
Night blindness, 281, 283
Nystagmus, 117

Ophthalmology, 1, 214
Ophthalmometer, 34, 60, 66
Ophthalmoscope, 23, 117, 160
Optic nerve, 89, 108, 111, 112,
   122, 127, 157
Optimums, 198

Pain, 133, 155, 202, 288
Palming, 123 (see also "Mem-
   ory")
Paralysis, 131
Parsons, 184
Patagonians, 2
Pearson, 256
Pessimums, 198
Pigmies, 3
Polyopia, 112, 149, 174, 178, 179,
   283
Presbyopia, 210

Pupil, 190, 214
Purkinje, 24, 25

Ray, 37
Reading, 192
Refraction, errors of (see also
   "Astigmatism," "Hyper-
   metropia," "Myopia")
   cause, 1, 14, 89, 106 (see
    also "production")
   occurrence, 5, 75, 98, 251,
    267, 285
   prevention, 1, 245, 285, 288
   production, 14, 38, 62, 75,
    89, 106, 114
   treatment, 1, 101, 112, 118,
    123, 136, 148, 159, 183,
    242, 246, 259, 270, 274
Refraction, variability of, 10,
   75, 85, 213, 215, 286, 287
Relaxation (see "Refraction,
   errors of, treatment")
Retina, 89, 109, 111, 114, 220
Retinoscope, 17, 110, 137
Rheumatism, 208
Risley, 253
Roosa, 210, 308
Rosenau, 4

Sanson, 29
Saturn, rings of, 121
Scheiner, 24
School-books, 192, 253
de Schweinitz, 36, 211
Sclera (see "Images, on scle-
   ra")
Scotomata, 177, 185, 186
Scott, 4
Sense, nerves of, 108
Shifting, 159
Sidler-Huguenin, 8, 82, 256
Snellen, 19
Snellen, jr., 69
Snellen test card, 19, 200, 242,
   244, 268, 287
Soldiers and sailors, 5, 284
Squint, 112, 117, 118, 221, 227,
   272
Steiger, 256
Stevens, 222

Strain, 89, 106, 115, 172, 178, 192, 257
Swinging, 159

Truth, 74
Tscherning, 27, 30, 252

Verhoeff, 184
Vision, defects of, 4, 264 (see also "Refraction, errors of, occurrence;" "Refraction, variability of")
    limits of, 104, 121
    military standards of, 5

Vision, primitive, 1, 2, 3, 6, 15, 16, 121, 267, 275
    standard of normal, 19, 123
Visual centers, 108, 123
Völkers, 29

Webster, 35
Whooping cough, 208
Woinow, 33
Worth, 222, 223, 225

Young, Dr. A. G., 193
Young, Dr. Thomas, 24, 30
    portrait, 28

www.ingramcontent.com/pod-product-compliance
Lightning Source LLC
Chambersburg PA
CBHW020243290326
41930CB00038B/157